PRACTICAL
Aromatherapy

PENNY RICH

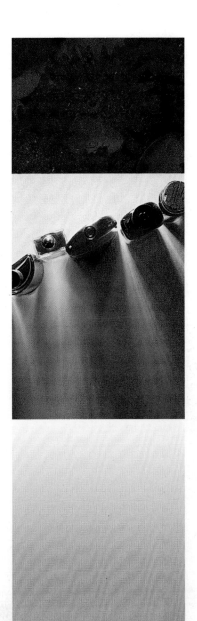

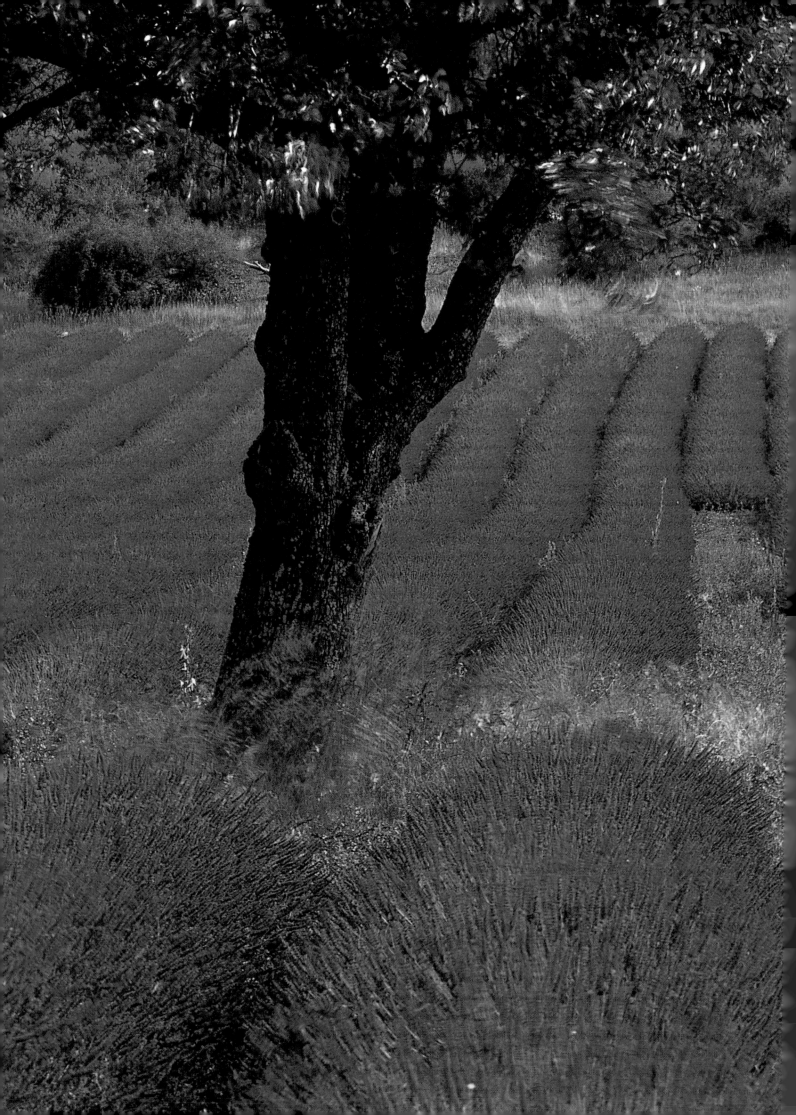

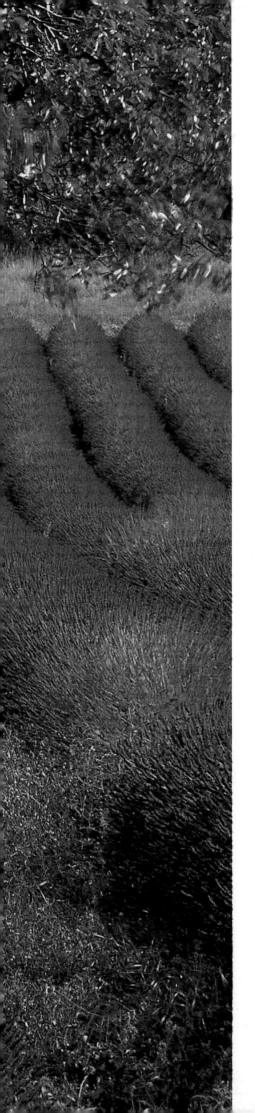

PRACTICAL

Aromatherapy

PENNY RICH

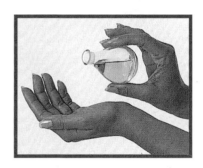

‖ •PARRAGON• ‖

First published in Great Britain in 1994 by
Parragon Book Service Ltd
Unit 13-17 Avonbridge Trading Estate
Atlantic Road, Avonmouth
Bristol BS11 9QD

This edition published in 1996

ISBN 0 75251 933 6

Editorial: Linda Doeser Publishing Services
Design and DTP: Kingfisher Design Services, London
Illustrator: Wayne Ford
Step-by-step photography: Susanna Price

Printed in Great Britain

CONTENTS

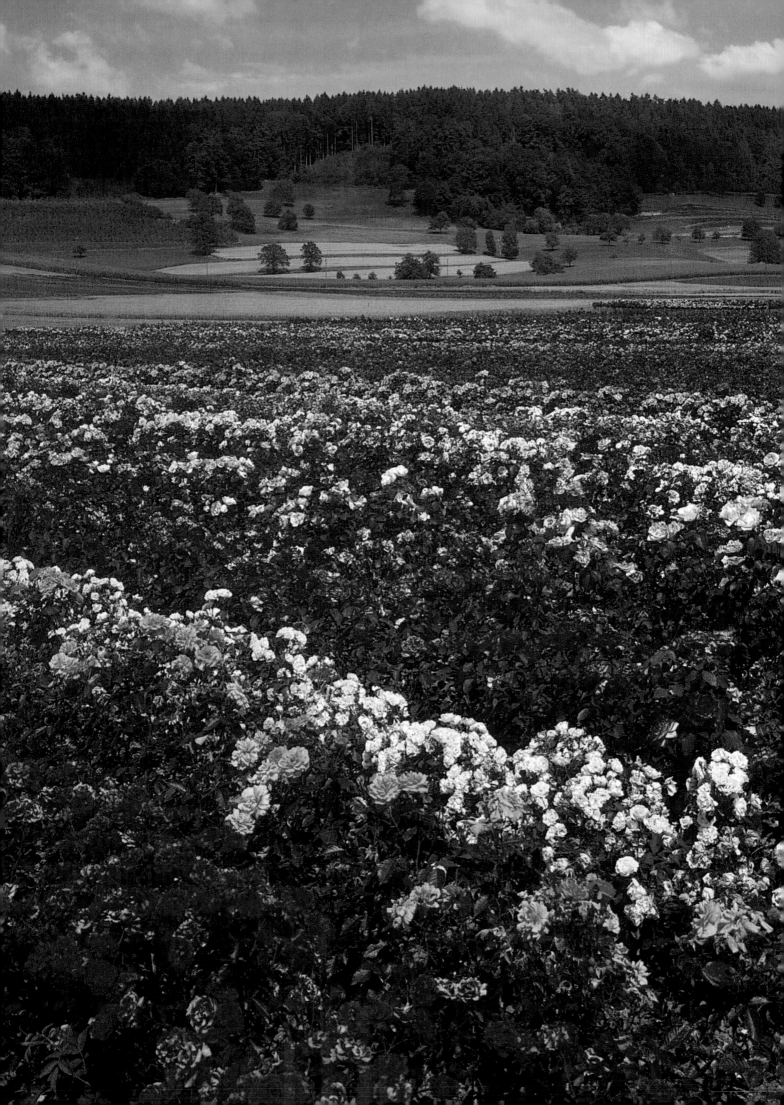

WHAT IS AROMATHERAPY?

Aromatherapy is a modern name for the ancient knowledge of healing and improving health using fragrant, natural ingredients. These ingredients, called essential oils, are found in herbs, plants, flowers, fruits and the bark, roots or resin of some trees.

Essential oils give the aroma to the plant, but they also contain dozens of complex chemicals that seem to do everything from beautifying skin or speeding healing to putting you to sleep or numbing a headache.

Even if you think you have never come across these oils before, all of us are affected by them each day. Every time you peel an orange, the essential oil squirts out of the tiny pockets in the peel and, because it is so volatile, instantly evaporates into the air releasing its bitter-sweet, tangy, citrus smell. And whether you notice or not, the orange oil has a refreshing but relaxing effect.

When you take flowers to someone who is ill in hospital you are using aromatherapy to help them feel better. The essential oils that give the smell to a bouquet of jasmine, roses, geranium, and lavender, for instance, all contain chemicals that relax the nervous system and instantly improve spirits.

When you use pure essential oils though, the beneficial properties are more concentrated, and have a greater effect on both mind and body than you get from just sniffing a bunch of flowers. So learning how you can use these essential oils will give you the means to be healthier, happier and more in control of every area of your life.

WHAT IS AN ESSENTIAL OIL?

Essential oils are so complex and magical that no one really knows what they are. Romantics and enthusiasts say they are the life force of a plant, similar to the human spirit. Researchers say they are a mixture of organic compounds, such as ketones, terpenes, esters, alcohols, aldehydes, and hundreds of other molecules, many too small or complex to classify under a microscope.

(Left) The sweet smell of roses has an uplifting, positive effect.

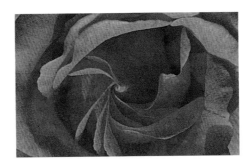

What they do, rather than what they are, is much easier to understand. Because the molecules of essential oils are so minute and so quick to evaporate, they penetrate human skin and enter the bloodstream and organs, before eventually being excreted. Scientists have found that the same oils gather in the same parts of the body time and time again, within a few hours of being massaged into skin. This is what makes them unique and so therapeutic, since very few things can actually penetrate human skin.

The fact that essential oils have healing properties is beyond doubt. Today, scientists studying botanicals find more and more vital ingredients in nature rather than in testtubes. For instance the painkiller aspirin comes from the willow tree, the Australian tea-tree contains a germ-killer a dozen times more effective than carbolic, and good old carrots are full of beta-carotene, now shown to be an important weapon in the battle against cancer.

The more that researchers study plants and their properties, the more benefits they discover from every organic compound in nature. Everything, it seems, is there for a reason. The most interesting discovery of all though, is that the latest research confirms the herbal traditions healers have practised for centuries.

ANCIENT AROMATICS

Since the beginning of life on Earth, mankind has had to experiment with plants to find out which were edible and which were fatal. Along the way, some were put aside for magic or medicine, and it is from these that the many folk remedies evolved.

By the time most of the ancient civilisations were thriving, therapeutic use of essential oils was part of everyday life. The Egyptians, in 4500 BC, used myrrh and cedarwood oils for embalming and, 6500 years later, perfectly preserved mummies are proof of their skills. Modern research has shown that cedarwood contains a natural fixative and myrrh has strong anti-bacterial and antiseptic agents, which explains why most mummies look so good for their age.

The Egyptians were the first to distil plants in order to extract their essential oils. They used them medicinally, in religious ceremonies, as beautifying skin and face potions and perfumes, as well as for embalming. Oils were so highly

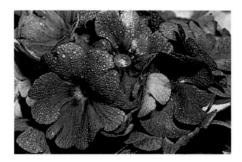

prized they were offered to the gods. The high priests recorded the oils'
therapeutic uses and known properties on papyrus scrolls, along with the secret
recipes that used them. Their knowledge was so accurate that it
makes up the basis of modern aromatherapy.

The Romans, on the other hand, used essential oils for giving pleasure as much as for
curing pain, and had leisurely, perfumed baths and massages every day.
Emperor Nero's love of orgies, feasts and fragrances is legendary. His most favourite
oil was rose because it cured headaches, indigestion and lifted the spirits,
thereby making it possible for him to keep on partying. Another Roman favourite was
chamomile, used to treat skin complaints and help heal wounds, and now
known to contain azulene, a natural anti-inflammatory agent, which is
why it has such a rejuvenating effect on skin.

In Greece, India, China and Arabia the use of aromatics thrived. But it wasn't until the
12th century that perfumery and herbalism spread to Europe. By the time
of the Great Plague in 1665, it was so well established that Londoners burnt bundles
of lavender, cedar and cypress in the streets, and carried posies of the
same plants as their only defence against infectious disease. And it undoubtedly saved
thousands of lives, since these plants all contain powerful antiseptic agents.

Plants were used to make all medicines and remedies until the turn of the century,
Herbalists and apothecaries dispensed infusions, ointments and powders
for everything from hair loss to impotence. But 'modern' medicine soon took over,
with pharmaceutical scientists creating tiny, magical pills which
made many of the natural remedies seem primitive and old-fashioned. By the 1960s,
the world focused on the advances made in surgery, hospitals and
doctoring while research into herbal cures took second place.

MODERN AROMATHERAPY

Although it is based on more than 6000 years' knowledge, the term 'Aromathérapie'
was first used only 65 years ago by a French chemist named Gattefossé.
His family owned a perfumery business. One day, while working in the laboratory,
Gattefossé badly burnt his hand and plunged it into a vat of lavender
essential oil. When the burn healed quickly without blistering, Gattefossé began his
lifelong obsession - studying the therapeutic properties of plant oils.

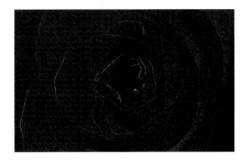

And so, modern aromatherapy was born. Since then, many enthusiasts, such as Dr Jean Valnet, have taken research further. Valnet used oils extensively to treat wounded soldiers during World War II. But it was a French woman biochemist, Marguerite Maury, who developed the method of diluting and applying essential oils by massage that we know as aromatherapy today.

It is only since the 1980s that modern aromatherapy has come of age. Biochemists have recently isolated dozens of ingredients in essential oils that account for the amazing properties they have. And now that the folk remedies have been substantiated by scientific fact, aromatherapy has become widely accepted and more popular than ever before.

ESSENTIAL DETAILS

Essential oils come from different parts of plants. In some they seem to accumulate in the petals, in others the roots, rinds, stalks, seeds, sap, nuts, leaves or bark. Sandalwood oil gathers in the heart wood of the tree, but only once the tree is 40 years old. Jasmine is most concentrated in the petals on the night when the flowers are one day old, so they need to be hand picked before dawn to give the best oil.

Rose is the rarest and most expensive of all essential oils. Two tons of fresh petals in full bloom yield a mere one kg (two pounds) of essential oil. The humble orange tree on the other hand produces three oils - neroli from the blossoms, petitgrain from the leaves and orange oil from the fruit rind - each of which has its own distinct properties.

The quality of an essential oil can vary from year to year, just like the vintage of a fine wine. Altitude and soil affect quality, as much as climate and the exact moment of harvest. Picking the raw ingredient is only the first consideration, for if they are left too long or not extracted using the best possible method, the essential oils might end up being inferior.

It is important to buy pure essential oils from a reputable source, as inferior quality or prediluted ones may have lost potency. Fortunately, with the increased interest in aromatherapy it is now possible to buy fine oils from specialist beauty outlets, mail order companies and health food shops throughout the Western world. Your nearest Aromatherapy Association will be able to offer guidance.

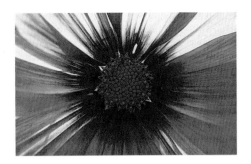

METHODS OF EXTRACTION

The biggest surprise with essential oils is that they are not oily at all. The majority are light liquids that don't dissolve in water but evaporate instantly when exposed to the air. They come in many shades: patchouli oil is plum-coloured, chamomile is clear blue, violet is forest green, sage is pale lime, sandalwood a golden yellow and geranium is colourless.

The liquid is held in tiny sacs somewhere on the living plant. Extracting it before it escapes into the air can be very complicated. The easiest and least expensive method is to turn the raw materials into steam and distil the oil. The most time-consuming and labour-intensive way is to press the flowers into trays of fat and replace them with fresh blooms every day for up to three months until the fat is saturated with essential oil. Citrus fruit peel is pressed by machine or hand and the oil is collected in sponges below. Plant resins are usually mixed with a solvent and alcohol to help separate the essential oil from the gum resin.

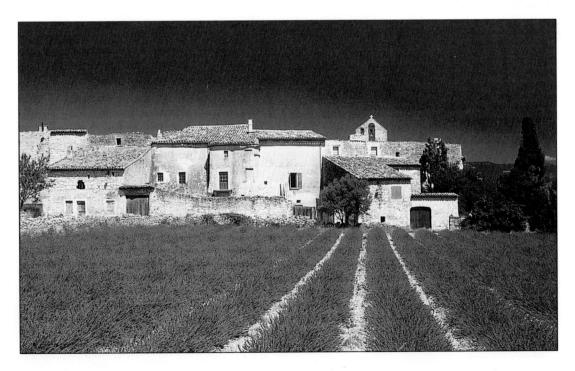

(Above) Lavender under cultivation in Provence, France.

11

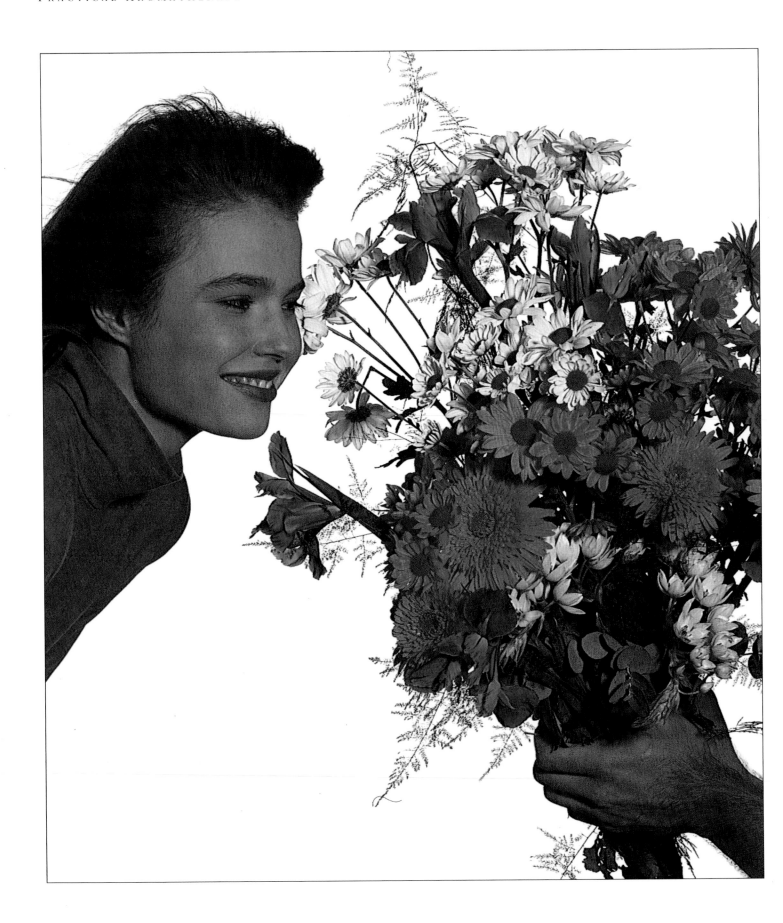

T E S T   Y O U R   S C E N T U A L I T Y

Today we rely on our sense of smell less than ever before. Once it led us to food, warned us of enemies or danger and guided us to the campfires of friends. Now, most of us have let our sense of smell slip to the point where we only notice particularly pleasant or offensive smells. Everything in between is ignored by the nose. However, we still react subconsciously to those smells. Freshly cooked food triggers saliva when you're hungry, just as freshly cut grass relaxes you when you are stressed.

This instinctive response to smell is what aromatherapy, which has become one of the most exciting new areas of research for industry, is based on. In France, perfume manufacturers are now creating 'mood' fragrances to make the wearer feel and smell better in one go. In America, car manufacturers are currently researching air-conditioning systems to time-release essential oils and keep motorists alert at the wheel. In Japan an alarm clock that pre-releases fragrance so you wake in a good mood is available. And in the United Kingdom relaxing odours are given to patients in hospital to prepare them for therapy. Developments like these are soon going to make our sense of smell more important once again.

There are more than 10,000 different odours that the human nose can smell, but most of us can only recognise a tenth of them because we have become so lazy. Happily, smells, like many other things, can be relearnt and memorised. All you have to do is train your nose to be aware of the different aromas it encounters.

To help you, here are two simple tests which use common household ingredients and will tell you (1) how good your sense of smell is, and (2) which essential oils you will like best.

For the first test, you need to wear a blindfold and have a friend or partner assist you; the second you can do alone.

(Left) Scents can induce a state of harmony and well-being.

— 1 —
THE SNIFF AND TELL TEST

Using the chart below, get your friend to choose any ten items that you have in the house. It is important that you don't know the ones selected, so wear your blindfold, and no peeping.

Your friend must cut any fruit, crush fresh (but not dried) herbs and open jars, bottles or tubes, then, one by one, hold each item about three inches away from the tip of your nose for up to 30 seconds, while you try to guess what it is.

If you get five or more items correct, you have an above-average sense of smell. But don't rest on your laurels. Keep practising until you score ten out of ten.

— 2 —
THE FRAGRANCE FAMILY TEST

Again, using the chart below, choose three items from each category (three floral, three citrus, three green, etc). Mix them up and smell them randomly, putting the ones you like on one side and the ones you dislike on another. It helps if you keep your eyes closed while you sniff, as this will help you to concentrate on the smell rather than what you see.

Then work out which fragrance categories you liked the most smells from. These are the categories you naturally prefer. For example, you might like citrus and green more than floral, woody and spicy). The most common essential oils are listed under each of the fragrance categories on page 45.

Most good suppliers stock 40 or more oils, so when you start buying them restrict your initial choice to the categories you instinctively prefer.

USING ESSENTIAL OILS

Essential oils give pleasure with their wonderful smells, improve health and well-being with their magic ingredients, and can be used in dozens of ways throughout your home. And no matter how you use them, they don't need any special equipment or fancy preparation. It can be as simple as unscrewing the bottle and breathing in.

To show what an important part essential oils can play in your life, here are some suggestions for the most beneficial ways of using them.

GREEN	CITRUS	FLORAL	SPICY	WOODY/BALSAMIC
basil	lemon	roses	nutmeg	tea
mint	orange	lavender	cloves	peanut butter
rosemary	lime	lilies	ginger	coffee
clary sage	tangerine	jasmine	mustard	aftershave
thyme	marmalade	honey	gin	pencil shavings
marjoram	disinfectant	peach	sherry	burnt toast
melon		honeysuckle	cinnamon	wax polish
celery		perfume	peppercorns	leather
toothpaste		face cream	coriander	vinegar
white wine				

14

Massage

Massage is the most common way of using essential oils (see page 105). Some would say it is the most pleasurable, combining as it does, the senses of touch and smell. It is also the most therapeutic method as essential oils are diluted in a carrier oil, like sunflower, and rubbed directly into the skin. Massage has two further bonuses: it stimulates the circulation enabling the oils to disperse rapidly around the body, and the warmth of the skin-on-skin friction makes oils smell stronger, so you get quicker therapeutic benefits to both mind and body.

Baths

The most relaxing way to use essential oils is to add them to your bath. You only need a few drops of oil (see page 72) in a tub of hot water to get the full benefits. The two main ones are that you have steam and warmth to evaporate the oils and intensify the aroma, and water to soften skin and speed up oil absorption. All you have to do is lie back and soak for 15 minutes.

Room Vaporisers

These provide a way of warming essential oils so that their aromas spread quickly to scent a room (see page 96). Vaporisers are little pots with a bowl-shaped bottom to hold a candle, and a saucer-shaped top to hold some water enriched with a few drops of essential oil. The candle heats the water and the oil rapidly vaporises and disperses through the air. You can achieve the same effect by putting a saucer of warm water on top of a hot radiator and adding a few drops of oil to the water. You can also buy ring burners. They hold a few drops of essential oil and sit around a lightbulb, which heats the liquid and dispersed the oil's fragrance.

Beauty Treatments

Some essential oils are great skin soothers, some heal skin quickly, others rejuvenate mature complexions or reduce oiliness, and some just smell divine on your face. They make wonderful beauty treatments (see page 85) from cleansers and masks to facials and moisturisers, all of which make you look good and feel good in one go.

Body Moisturisers

Essential oils penetrate skin so rapidly and deeply they make excellent, inexpensive and indulgent body moisturisers (see page 77). You can mix them in any combination, for their aroma, their treatment effect, or both, and add them to a rich carrier oil, such as apricot, jojoba or peach. Or simply add a few drops of essential oil to the cheapest, simplest body moisturising lotion you can buy.

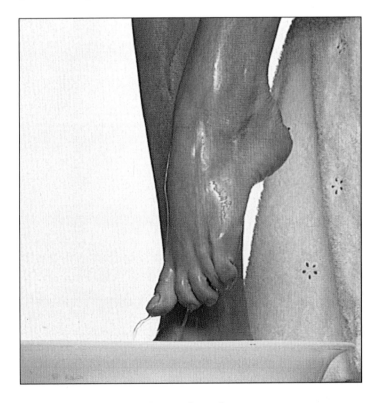

Footbaths

For the most sensual footbath, add a few drops of essential oil (see page 75) to a basin of water then sit back and soak your toes. You can add oils for their smell alone, or oils that will refresh tired feet, boost the circulation of cold feet, soothe aches, or help reduce perspiration.

Room Sprays

For a therapeutic air freshener (see page 97) using your own favourite fragrances, mix a few drops of essential oil with water in a pump-action spray bottle. Shake well before each use.

Air Purifier

One of the easiest ways to scent your whole house is to add your favourite essential oil to the dust bag of your vacuum cleaner (see page 99). As air is blown out, the oil will scent the room you are cleaning. If you want to use different aromas regularly, place the drops of oil on a cotton-wool ball beside the internal exit filter of your cleaner. This makes it easier to change fragrances.

Pot Pourri

To make your own pot pourri, add a few drops (see page 97) of a broad mix of floral, spicy and citrus essential oils to a bowl of dried flowers, herbs, grasses or seed pods. Then cover the bowl and leave it for a short time before tossing the dried flowers and stirring them so that they absorb the aromas. The pot pourri will scent your room up to six weeks.

Household Cleansers

Some of the most antiseptic essential oils make excellent natural household cleansers (see page 99). Pour a few drops on a damp cloth to wipe over work surfaces or rubbish bins. Or add to a bucket of warm water to clean floors, bathrooms or kitchens. You'll find they are inexpensive, non-chemical and have a better smell than most shop-bought cleansers.

Insect Repellent

Some essential oils are powerful natural insecticides (see page 103). Add a few drops of essential oil to a damp cloth and wipe inside wardrobes, around window frames or apply a few drops of oil directly onto the hems of curtains.

Deodorisers

Deodorising essential oils (see page 99) are good at getting rid of bacteria or viruses. To disinfect the air of a sickroom, burn oils in a vaporiser. Leave a few drops on a cotton ball inside your wardrobe and laundry basket, or rub over the insoles of shoes to stop odour. A couple of drops on the inside, underarm seam of shirts or jumpers have the same effect.

Wood Fires

Pour a few drops of your favourite essential oil onto wood about 15 minutes before lighting the fire (see pages 97-98). The heat will release the fragrance throughout the room. This is particularly good at Christmas and other family occasions if you use something special like orange, ginger and sandalwood.

Bedtime Treatments

Apply a few drops of your favourite oil to a tissue before going to bed and leave it beside your pillow so you inhale it while you sleep (see page 96). You can use oils that relax you, oils with aphrodisiac properties, oils that treat insomnia, colds or headache, and oils that boost confidence or lift bad moods. For daytime, apply to a handkerchief, as the aroma lingers longer on fabric.

Inhalation

Inhaling essential oils is one of the best ways to treat coughs or colds. Add a few drops of oil to a bowl of boiling water, cover your head with a towel, bend over the bowl and inhale deeply for several minutes. Steam also opens the pores and lets oils enter the skin, so it is a good way to enjoy a facial (see page 92) to deep-cleanse, moisturise or to brighten a dull complexion.

Hot Poultices

This is an ideal way to use essential oils to relieve muscular pain and reduce chest congestion (see page 100). Add a few drops of essential oil to a bowl of very

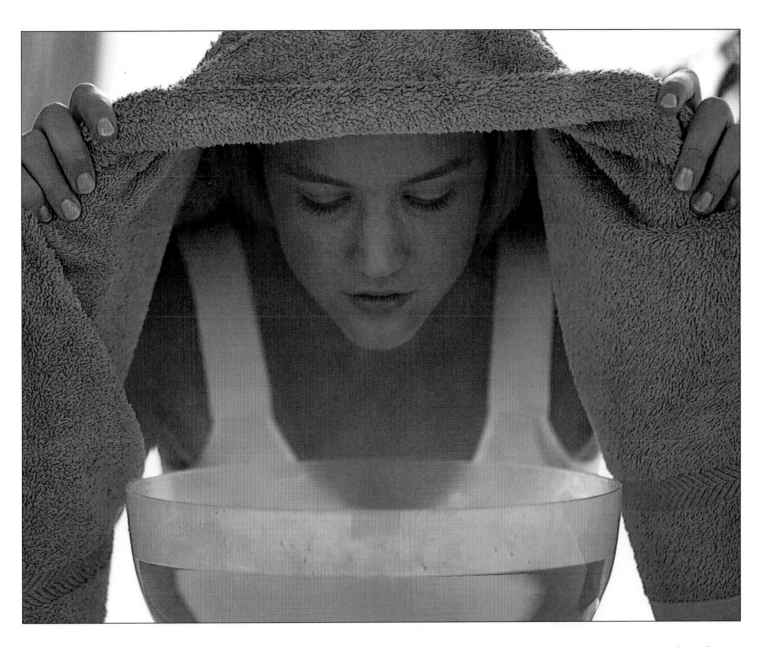

hot water and, wearing rubber gloves, dip in a folded cotton cloth or flannel. Then squeeze out excess water and place it over the effected area until it has cooled to blood temperature. Reheat and repeat the process.

(Above) Inhaling oils with steam gives maximum benefit in minimum time.

Cold Compresses

Use these to soothe inflammation (see page 102) and reduce fever. Follow the same procedure as for poultices, but use ice-cold water rather than hot.

Hair Care

Some essential oils work wonders on dull, lifeless or thinning hair (see page 56). You can add a few drops of oil to a mild, fragrance-free shampoo. Or mix it with olive oil and rub through the scalp as a weekly, deep-conditioning treatment.

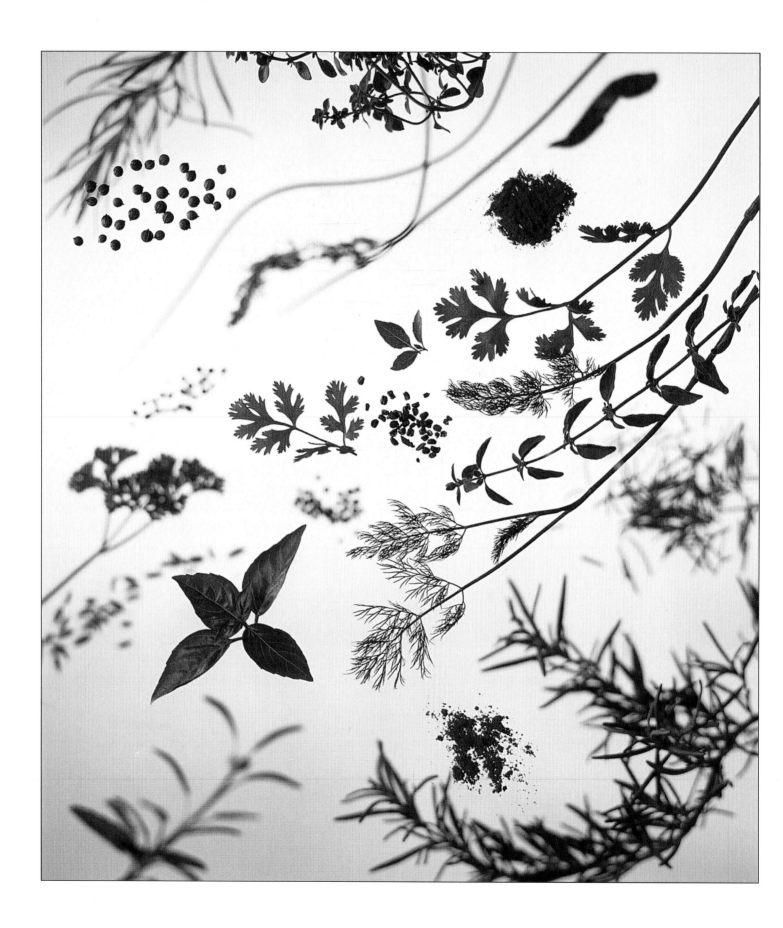

THE A-Z DIRECTORY
of
ESSENTIAL OILS

The Directory has been compiled to give you all the information you could possibly need to know about essential oils, their properties and the benefits they yield. It also guides you to the oils you, personally, will like best. It takes the guesswork out of combining oils, by showing which blend well together. And it tells you exactly which oils work best for particular health or lifestyle problems.

HOW TO USE THE DIRECTORY

You can use it from any reference point you have. If you want to see what lavender oil does, turn to the alphabetical list of the 48 most common essential oils (see page 20); it includes details of where each oil is from, the herbal traditions, properties, aromatherapy actions, the most common home uses and any safety warnings that must be heeded.

If you have a headache and can't be bothered reading through all 48 essential oils to find out which works best, turn to the Index of Common Problems (see page 52) for an alphabetical list of problems, from acne to wrinkles, with a list of the essential oils that will help resolve them.

If you want to assess the overall usefulness of a particular oil, turn to the at-a-glance chart (see page 50), which summarises the things it does best.

If you are not sure whether the little recipe of essential oils you are mixing up will be sweet-smelling or just sickly-sweet, use the chart that shows which oils blend well together (see page 46).

(Left) Flowers, fruit, seeds, roots, leaves or stems may yield oils.

AMBRETTE SEED • ABELMOSCHUS MOSCHATUS

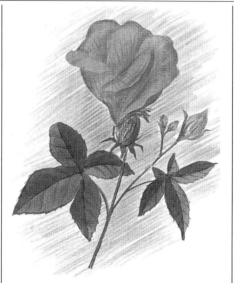

EXTRACTION
Oil is extracted from the musky, kidney-shaped, fully ripened seeds. The evergreen shrub grows well in India, and is cultivated in the West Indies, China and Indonesia.

HERBAL TRADITION
Ambrette seed is ground and used as a spice in the East, and as a musk substitute in perfumery. Traditionally, it cures cramp, indigestion, acidity and other stomach complaints, and treats headaches and nerves.

PROPERTIES
The essential oil has a rich, musky smell and has both relaxing and stimulating properties. It is warming and calming and said to be an aphrodisiac.

ACTIONS
In aromatherapy, it is effective for anxiety, depression, fatigue or other stress-related conditions. It is also good for cramps, muscular aches and poor circulation.

HOME USE
Massage, baths, inhalation, compress. A few drops on a tissue can clear your head, whether you're suffering from a cold or mental fatigue, and relieve headaches or any nausea, from travel to morning sickness. Four drops in a basin will refresh tired feet. Use sparingly for massage or in the bath.

WARNING
Ambrette seed oil is perfectly safe for home use as long as it is diluted before application.

ANGELICA • ANGELICA ARCHANGELICA

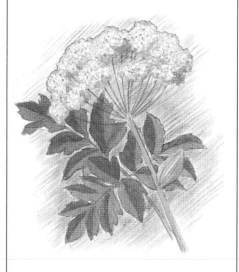

EXTRACTION
Oil is extracted from the root, fruit or seed of the plant. It is grown in Belgium, Hungary, Germany and is a native of Europe.

HERBAL TRADITION
Angelica is best known as the green, candied stem used to decorate cakes. Traditionally the root was chewed and burnt to ward off infection during 14th- and 15th-century plagues and to cure coughs or indigestion.

PROPERTIES
The essential oil has an earthy, peppery, musky smell. It is a good expectorant, an excellent digestive, and helps with rheumatic conditions, indigestion, flatulence and colic.

ACTIONS
In aromatherapy, it is a germ-killer, excellent for coughs and colds, 'flu, muscular aches and rheumatism. It has a calming effect on the digestion and is warming and relaxing.

HOME USE
Massage, baths, inhalation, compress. A few drops on a tissue clears a blocked nose and when inhaled with steam it relieves the congestion of a chesty or smoker's cough. Five drops in the bath, or mixed with two tablespoons of carrier oil and massaged in, will speed the healing of cuts and bruises, relieve indigestion and soothe aching joints or muscles.

WARNING
The root oil is photo-toxic, so avoid exposure to sunshine after use or it may cause skin irritations. Not to be used during pregnancy.

20

BASIL • OCIMUM BASILICUM

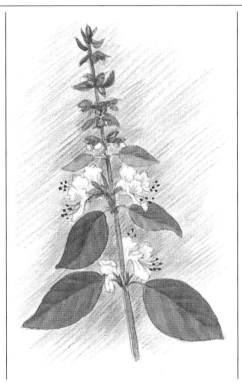

EXTRACTION
Oil is extracted from the flowering sweet basil. Today it is grown commercially throughout Europe, the Mediterranean, Pacific Islands and in America.

HERBAL TRADITION
Basil has been thought of as an aphrodisiac for centuries and featured heavily in most diets. It was once thought to ward off evil spirits and is still worn tucked in the hat to scare away insects in Mediterranean climates.

PROPERTIES
The essential oil has a very high proportion of camphor and a warm, aromatic, sweet-spicy smell. It is a refreshing, light and uplifting tonic.

ACTIONS
In aromatherapy, it is used for nervous insomnia, anxiety and tiredness, insect bites, headaches, poor circulation and muscular aches or sprains.

HOME USE
Massage, baths, inhalation. A few drops on a tissue clears the head. Diluted with massage oil, it can be rubbed in to relieve insect bites or aches and pains. And the smell of sweet basil in the bath will lift your spirits.

WARNING
Basil is potent and may cause skin irritation in some people, so always use cautiously. Avoid during pregnancy.

BAY, WEST INDIAN • PIMENTA RACEMOSA

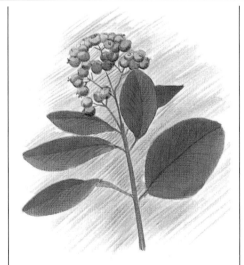

EXTRACTION
The essential oil is extracted from the dried leaves and berries of the bay rum tree. A native of South America, it is now grown in Barbados, Jamaica and throughout the West Indies.

HERBAL TRADITION
West Indian bay leaves have traditionally been steeped in rum to make hair tonic. Though the Victorians thought it cured hair loss, it is now known to be mildly antiseptic and helps treat greasy hair or flaky scalps.

PROPERTIES
The essential oil has a woody, masculine, clove-like smell and is both warming and stimulating. It is antiseptic and has astringent properties.

ACTIONS
In aromatherapy, it is excellent as a scalp stimulant, removing grease from hair and bringing blood to the skin surface. It is also good for poor circulation, cellulite or muscular aches.

HOME USE
Massage, inhalation, compress, poultice. It is best used well-diluted with a friction massage, to increase the circulation-boosting effects, particularly on the scalp, across stiff, tense shoulders, directly on aching muscles or areas of cellulite, and to warm winter-chilled hands or feet. It can be inhaled with steam to relieve nose, throat or chest infections.

WARNING
Bay should be used in moderation only as it can irritate the mucous membrane. Its main constituent, eugenol, can corrode metal so always store in a dark, glass bottle.

BERGAMOT • CITRUS AURANTIUM BERGAMIA

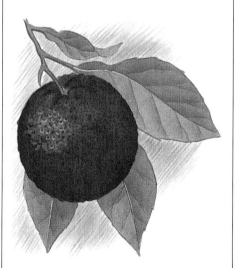

EXTRACTION
Oil is extracted from the peel of the nearly ripe, bitter orange fruit. Today it is grown commercially in Morocco southern Italy, Sicily and parts of Africa.

HERBAL TRADITION
Bergamot has been used since the 16th century in southern Europe to counter fever. It is bergamot that gives Earl Grey tea its flavour, and is a common fragrance and fixative in cosmetics, toiletries and suntanning products.

PROPERTIES
The essential oil is uplifting, refreshing and antiseptic. It has a fresh, subtle, spicy lemon, smell with a warm, balsamic undertone.

ACTIONS
In aromatherapy, it is used to treat depression, melancholy, tiredness, irritability, stress, acne and greasy skins. It is a good deodorant and will help kill germs in the home.

HOME USE
Massage, baths, inhalation. Because of its wonderful smell, destressing effect and antiseptic properties, place a few drops in a saucer of hot water on top of a radiator to freshen a room. It may be inhaled directly from a tissue for emotional upset or negative moods. Use it in moderation, a maximum of five drops, for massage or in a bath to lift your spirits.

WARNING
Bergamot oil can irritate skin, especially if it is subsequently exposed to sunlight. It is safe for home use, if well diluted.

BIRCH (WHITE) • BETULA ALBA

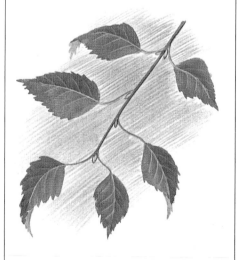

EXTRACTION
Oil is extracted from the leaf buds and bark of the white birch tree. It is grown in northern Russia, Germany, Sweden and Finland.

HERBAL TRADITION
Birch has been used for centuries as a treatment for skin complaints and arthritic or rheumatic conditions. Scandinavians hang small bundles of the leafy branches in their saunas in order to create a fragrant steam which will deep cleanse the skin and boost the circulation.

PROPERTIES
The essential oil is soothing, anti-inflammatory, antiseptic and diuretic. It has a woody, leathery, warm smell.

ACTIONS
In aromatherapy, it is excellent for dry skin, dandruff and eczema, as well as fungal infections. It also helps break down cellulite and stop fluid retention.

HOME USE
Massage, baths. Diluted with a carrier oil, massage into the thighs, buttocks and tummy to reduce the 'bloat' of PMT or help break down stubborn cellulite. Massage it on areas of extra-dry skin or add a few drops to a warm bath. And a few drops in a hot footbath will soothe fungal infections such as athlete's foot.

WARNING
Birch essential oil is perfectly safe for home use as long as it is diluted before application.

CAMPHOR (WHITE) • CINNAMOMUM CAMPHORA

EXTRACTION
Oil is extracted from the wood, root stumps and young branches of the evergreen camphor tree. It is a native of China, Taiwan and Japan, but is now grown as far afield as India and California.

HERBAL TRADITION
Camphor has traditionally been worn around the neck to ward off evil spirits, infectious diseases and to strengthen the heart. It has long been used as an insecticide, particularly in moth balls.

PROPERTIES
The essential oil contains terpenic ketone, which is why it has such hot, pungent fumes. It is good for sprains or muscular aches and pains.

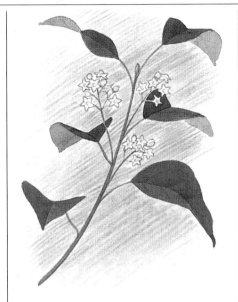

ACTIONS
In aromatherapy, it is good for softening tight, aching muscles, relieving minor sprains, or soothing a stiff neck. It also repels most insects.

HOME USE
Massage. Camphor should be used sparingly and must be well diluted for massaging directly into aching or painful muscles. Add a few drops to a cotton ball, or the hem of curtains or blinds, for an excellent insect repellent, particularly for flies and moths.

WARNING
Camphor oil fumes are potent and should not be inhaled by asthmatics. It is safe for massage if well diluted and applied to specific areas, rather than all over the body.

CEDARWOOD (ATLAS) • CEDRUS ATLANTICA

EXTRACTION
Oil is extracted from the wood of the evergreen coniferous tree. Originally from Lebanon, today the finest essential oil comes from Morocco.

HERBAL TRADITION
Cedars are thought to offer longevity and so the trees have traditionally been grown in graveyards, and the oil it yields used for embalming in ancient Egypt, and as incense in the East and Tibet. It is said to cure baldness and skin complaints such as eczema.

PROPERTIES
The essential oil has a woody smell, similar to lead-pencil shavings. It is stimulating, refreshing and has an astringent, tonic effect.

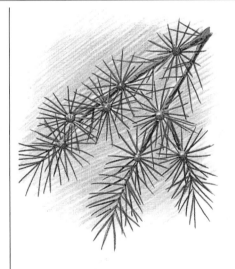

ACTIONS
In aromatherapy, it is good for dandruff, thinning hair, dermatitis, rashes, eczema, greasy skin and acne. It also helps with any stress-related symptoms.

HOME USE
Massage, baths. For dry skin conditions, dilute with oil or add a few drops to a simple moisturising cream, and massage in. For greasy skin conditions, add a few drops to a basin of boiling water and bend over it with a towel over your head for a steam facial. It also makes an excellent scalp-massage oil.

WARNING
Moroccan cedarwood is perfectly safe for home use as long as it is diluted before application. However, it is best avoided during pregnancy.

CHAMOMILE (GERMAN) • MATRICARIA RECUTITA

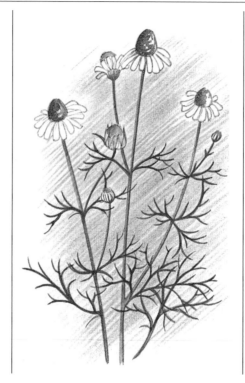

EXTRACTION
Oil is extracted from the freshly dried, daisy-like flowers. The plant is grown in eastern Europe and North America.

HERBAL TRADITION
Chamomile is one of the oldest British medicinal and beauty herbs. Traditionally, it was said to 'cure all agues'. It has been used most successfully to make blonde hair blonder, as an excellent disinfectant during World War II, and as a tea to treat insomniacs.

PROPERTIES
The essential oil is rich in azulene, a natural anti-inflammatory and healing agent. It has relaxing sedative benefits, and smells of apples and straw.

ACTIONS
In aromatherapy it is used for stress, sleeplessness, headaches, rashes, insect bites, burns, cuts, toothache and menstrual or menopausal problems.

HOME USE
Massage, baths, inhalation, compress. To relax after a hard day, add ten drops of oil to a warm bath. Diluted with a carrier oil, it can be massaged in, and used as a compress for headaches or menstrual problems. It is also an excellent household disinfectant.

WARNING
Chamomile essential oil is perfectly safe for home use as long as it is diluted before application.

CITRONELLA • CYMBOPOGON NARDUS

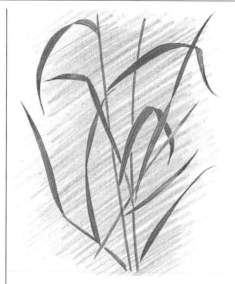

EXTRACTION
Oil is extracted from the freshly dried tropical grass. It grows naturally by the sea, and the best varieties come from Sri Lanka, Java and the Seychelles.

HERBAL TRADITION
Citronella leaves were traditionally used as a poultice for fever, pain and to speed healing. It was used in China for rheumatic pain, and throughout the East and Asia it is renowned as an excellent insect repellent.

PROPERTIES
The essential oil is strongly antiseptic and has an even stronger aromatic, lemony smell. It is good for aches and pains and has a powerful deodorising effect.

ACTIONS
In aromatherapy, it is effective for rheumatic problems, sprains or muscular aches. It is an excellent antiseptic and germicide and increases mental alertness.

HOME USE
Baths, inhalation, compress. A few drops on a tissue can clear your head, or burn the oil in a room to kill germs and freshen the air. As a poultice, it soothes aches and is excellent at reducing excessive perspiration. A few drops on your bedding will keep insects away, and applying the diluted oil directly on mosquito or other bites will stop the itching and act as an antiseptic.

WARNING
Citronella is perfectly safe for home use as long as it is well diluted before application. However, it is best avoided during pregnancy.

Cypress • *Cupressus sempervirens*

EXTRACTION
Oil is extracted from the freshly picked leaves, twigs and cones of the evergreen tree. It is native to the Mediterranean but is now cultivated throughout Europe and North America.

HERBAL TRADITION
The Cypress tree was prized by the ancient Greeks. It was used medicinally and to make sarcophagi by the Egyptians. It has a tradition of easing internal bleeding and is now known to be a good vasco-constrictor.

PROPERTIES
The essential oil has a warm, woody, balsamic smell and a refreshing, invigorating effect. It is astringent, antiseptic and boosts the circulation.

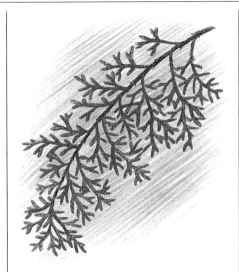

ACTIONS
In aromatherapy, it is excellent for menstrual or menopausal problems, varicose or broken veins, fluid retention or cellulite, and to calm a persistent cough.

HOME USE
Massage, baths, inhalation, compress, poultice. Diluted with a carrier oil, it makes a good abdomen-to-thigh massage for fluid retention, a warming hand or foot massage, and an excellent leg massage for varicose veins. As a poultice, it helps with menstrual aches or swelling, and a few drops sprinkled on a pillow will stop coughing.

WARNING
Cypress is perfectly safe for home use as long as it is diluted before application.

Eucalyptus • *Eucalyptus globulus*

EXTRACTION
Oil is extracted from the twigs and leaves of the Blue Gum tree. A native of Australia, it is now grown in California, Spain and Portugal.

HERBAL TRADITION
Eucalyptus leaves were crushed and used by the Aborigines to heal wounds, fight infection and to relieve muscular pain. The wood was used on cooking fires to flavour food.

PROPERTIES
The essential oil has a distinctive, stimulating smell that clears the head and has been used in cough and cold remedies for decades. It is a powerful antiseptic that kills airborne germs and has a cooling effect on skin.

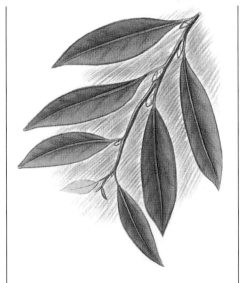

ACTIONS
In aromatherapy, it is an excellent decongestant for fever, flu, coughs, colds or sinus. It soothes muscular aches, sprains and pains and helps heal abrasions.

HOME USE
Massage, baths, inhalation, poultice. A few drops in a dish of hot water on a radiator will disinfect a room and make breathing easier at night, or use it for a chest massage, in a steamy bath, or on a hot, chest poultice. Diluted, it may be massaged into aching muscles for quick relief.

WARNING
Eucalyptus is perfectly safe for home use as long as it is diluted before application.

FENNEL • FOENICULUM VULGARE

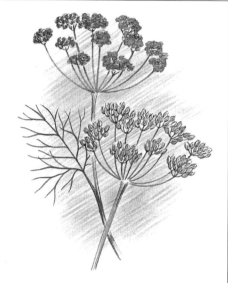

EXTRACTION
Oil is extracted from the crushed seeds of the sweet fennel plant. It is cultivated in France, Italy, Germany and parts of India.

HERBAL TRADITION
Fennel was used by the Egyptians, Chinese, Indians and Greeks to give long life, power, courage and strength. Traditionally it cures digestive problems, eye infections and increases milk flow for nursing mothers.

PROPERTIES
The essential oil has a sweet anise-like, peppery smell and is a good digestive, diuretic, tonic and antiseptic. It is a common ingredient in babies' gripe water.

ACTIONS
In aromatherapy, it is excellent for tummy ache, menstrual cramps, fluid retention, PMT, and tiredness – particularly the exhaustion you get from too much physical activity.

HOME USE
Massage, baths, inhalation, poultice, compress. A few drops in a warm bath will have an energising effect. Or add some directly to a tissue and inhale it for an instant pick-me-up. Dilute and massage it in, or apply it with a warm compress, for any digestive complaints or tummy problems.

WARNING
Sweet fennel is perfectly safe for home use if well diluted and used in moderation. It should not be used during pregnancy or by people with epilepsy.

FRANKINCENSE • BOSWELLIA CARTERI

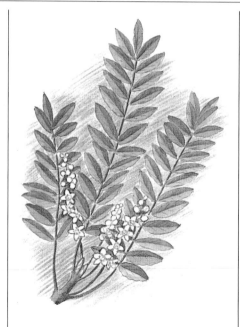

EXTRACTION
Oil is extracted from the gum resin of the tree. A native of Africa and the Middle East, the resin is now collected as far afield as China and then processed in Europe.

HERBAL TRADITION
Frankincense has been treasured for centuries and was burnt as the original incense to appease the gods, as well as being one of the three gifts to the infant Jesus. It was used by many cultures to treat almost all known ailments.

PROPERTIES
The essential oil has a warm, rich smell with a tang of lemon and woody camphor. It is relaxing, uplifting, calming and mildly antiseptic.

ACTIONS
In aromatherapy it is excellent for tiredness, grumpiness, negative moods, lack of confidence and emotional turmoil. It helps slow the breathing and has a calming effect.

HOME USE
Massage, baths, inhalation. Add a few drops to a massage oil to warm, relax and restore an overworked or overstressed body. Massage on the scalp and temples to relieve tension headaches. Inhale it directly or add it to a relaxing bath to remove stress and sweeten your mood.

WARNING
Frankincense is perfectly safe for home use as long as it is diluted before application.

GALBANUM • FEURLA GALBANIFLUA

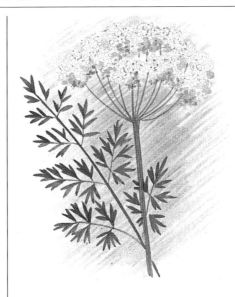

EXTRACTION
Oil is extracted from the gum resin of the giant fennel plant. It is grown commercially in southern Europe and North Africa.

HERBAL TRADITION
Galbanum has been used for centuries. The Egyptians used it for embalming, and the Hebrews as an anointing oil. It was also used as incense and in early cosmetics. Traditionally it heals, treats skin and digestive disorders and is calming.

PROPERTIES
The essential oil has a warm, woody, slightly melon-like smell. It is uplifting, soothing, calming and very refreshing and relaxing.

ACTIONS
In aromatherapy it is excellent for healing blemished, grazed or scarred skin. Also for stress, tension, fatigue, anxiety or nervous tension.

HOME USE
Massage, baths, inhalation. When mixed with more fragrant essential oils it makes a therapeutic facial massage for blemished skin or a deeply relaxing and restoring body massage or bath. Inhaled it has a tonic effect, but it is not the nicest smell on its own.

WARNING
Galbanum is perfectly safe for home use as long as it is well diluted before application.

GERANIUM • PELARGONIUM GRAVECLENS

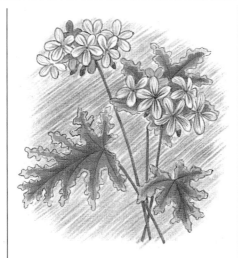

EXTRACTION
Oil is extracted from the fresh flowers, stalks and leaves of the perennial shrub. It is cultivated in Madagascar, Egypt, Spain, France, Italy, Russia and in the Congo.

HERBAL TRADITION
Geranium is now one of the commonest garden plants, blooming in a riot of colours and leaving its tangy, sweet aroma throughout the world. Traditionally, its close relative herb robert has been used in herbal medicine for centuries, but geranium oil was only discovered in the 1850s.

PROPERTIES
The essential oil has a rosy-sweet, lemon-and-mint smell and works as both a tonic and sedative on the nervous system. It is mildly antiseptic and a good skin-soother.

ACTIONS
In aromatherapy it is one of the most important oils – perfect to put you in a good mood, put you to sleep, give you energy or relax you totally. It is good for cuts, bruises, eczema, burns, acne, broken veins and mature or dry skin.

HOME USE
Massage, bath, inhalation, compress. Apply one drop directly on cuts or bruises to speed healing. Added to a hot bath, it is deeply relaxing and to a cooler one, energising. Mixed with a carrier oil it makes an excellent headache, neck and shoulder, or facial massage.

WARNING
Geranium is perfectly safe for home use.

GINGER • ZINGIBER OFFICINALIS

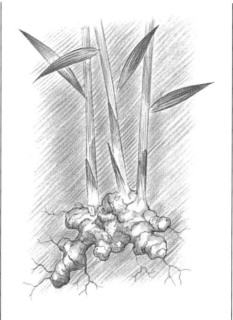

EXTRACTION
Oil is extracted from the dried root of the tropical herbaceous perennial. It is grown in the West Indies, Florida, Africa, India and Japan.

HERBAL TRADITION
Ginger has been used culinarily and medicinally by the ancient Egyptians, Greeks and Romans, and in India, China and Japan. In particular, it was recommended for stomach upsets and digestive disorders, but its warming effect also helps bring down a fever.

PROPERTIES
The essential oil has a lemony-pepper, woody-spice smell and has warming, stimulating, astringent and antiseptic properties.

ACTIONS
In aromatherapy it is good to boost the circulation, relieve a tight, chesty cough, tummy ache, tight muscles, stiffness, or exhaustion. The astringent and antiseptic actions make it effective to warm and freshen tired feet.

HOME USE
Massage, baths, inhalation, poultice. Inhale it from a tissue to clear the head and energise the body, and use it in poultices for stiff muscles, tummy ache or a cough. For bath and massage, it is particularly effective in cold weather because of its warming effect.

WARNING
Ginger is very potent so never apply it undiluted to skin, and use it in moderation for both bath and massage.

JASMINE • JASMINUM OFFICINALE

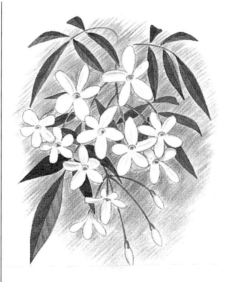

EXTRACTION
A single kilogram of oil is extracted from about eight million flowers, which are hand-picked before dawn – the reason jasmine oil is so expensive. It is grown in France, Egypt, Morocco, India and Italy.

HERBAL TRADITION
Jasmine has been prized, above all, for its scent which is romantic, rich, exotic and makes all who smell it feel better. It has long been used in toiletries and appears in most of the great, classic perfumes for its sensual note.

PROPERTIES
The essential oil is a deep red in colour and smells as fragrant as the flower – hence its value in perfumery. It is uplifting, relaxing and will leave you in a confident, optimistic and slightly euphoric mood. It is good for dry or sensitive skins and any aches or cramps.

ACTIONS
In aromatherapy it is excellent for any depression, stress, fatigue, irritability or apathy. It is also good for PMT and is an excellent skin-softener.

HOME USE
Massage, baths, inhalation, poultice, compress. Since jasmine mixes well with most other oils it is very good to add to any relaxing bath or massage. Add a few drops to a saucer of water and place on a radiator to make everyone in the room feel mellow.

WARNING
Jasmine essential oil is perfectly safe for home use as long as it is diluted before application.

JUNIPER • *JUNIPERUS COMMUNIS*

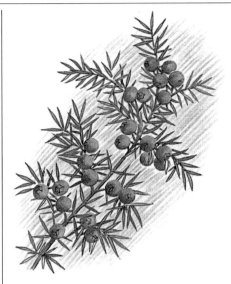

EXTRACTION
Oil is extracted from the fresh berries and needles of the evergreen Juniper tree. It is native to northern Europe and is grown commercially in Scandinavia, Italy, France, Spain and Canada.

HERBAL TRADITION
Juniper berries were used by the ancient Egyptians and Greeks to ward off infections; and in England juniper was burnt to scare off witches or demons. Today the berries are most commonly used to flavour gin.

PROPERTIES
The essential oil smells like pine, but with a hot, peppery edge. It is diuretic, antiseptic, uplifting but relaxing, and excellent for aches and pains.

ACTIONS
In aromatherapy, it is best for menstrual problems, fluid retention, cramps, slow circulation and cellulite.

It also has a toning effect on greasy skins or for acne, and a calming effect for the over-stressed.

HOME USE
Massage, baths, inhalation, compress, poultice. Diluted with a carrier oil, it is an ideal massage for rheumatism, aching joints or muscles or any PMT/menstrual problems. Add a few drops to the bath for a relaxing soak that will lift spirits. It is also a good germ-killer to burn in a sickroom.

WARNING
Juniper is perfectly safe for home use if well diluted but should never be used during pregnancy as it can trigger labour.

LAUREL • *LAUARUS NOBILIS*

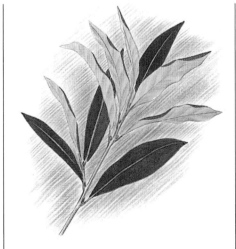

EXTRACTION
Oil is extracted from the leaves of the evergreen tree. It is cultivated in Italy, Greece, Balkan countries and France.

HERBAL TRADITION
The ancient Greeks believed that the laurel tree was protected by the gods. According to their mythology, the maiden Daphne was turned into a laurel tree to escape from Apollo. The Romans also prized it: Caesar wore a laurel crown after his victories in battle. Since classical times, it has been used as a culinary herb and powerful cure-all.

PROPERTIES
The essential oil has a strong medicinal smell with a warm, spicy edge. It is relaxing, warming, antiseptic and good for boosting the immune system.

ACTIONS
In aromatherapy it is useful for aches, pains, period cramps or fluid retention. If you constantly suffer from colds, flu or other viral infections, it is useful to strengthen resistance.

HOME USE
Massage, inhalation, poultice. Place some oil in a dish of hot water on a bedroom radiator to help dispel viral infections, or inhale the steam by bending over a basin of hot water. Use for massage to relieve PMT, fluid retention, aches or any chest complaints.

WARNING
Laurel should be used in moderation and well diluted as it can irritate sensitive skin. It should not be used during pregnancy.

LAVENDER • LAVANDULA AUGUSTIFOLIA

EXTRACTION
Oil is extracted from the flowering tips of the evergreen shrub. It is cultivated in southern Europe, and in countries as apart as Australia and Britain.

HERBAL TRADITION
Lavender was a favourite bathtime cleanser for the ancient Romans and has been used to speed healing. Since the 18th century it has been used in soap, perfumes, talc and pot-pourri.

PROPERTIES
The essential oil is one of the most commonly used. It is both relaxing and stimulating, a powerful antiseptic and healer, and it calms, refreshes, invigorates and lifts the spirits.

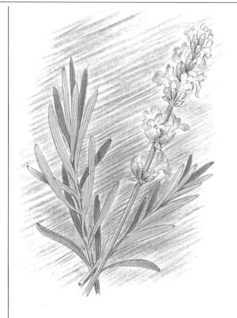

ACTIONS
In aromatherapy it is excellent for tension, tiredness or depression, skin problems and aches or pains. Because it is so gentle, it may be applied undiluted to burnt skin or insect bites, and is safe to use during pregnancy.

HOME USE
Massage, baths, inhalation, poultice, compress. A few drops in a hot bath will make you feel pleasantly drowsy and relieve anxiety. In a cool bath, it will refresh and energise. Inhale a few drops from a tissue to clear the head and lift the spirits. In massage, it is good for tense muscles or mental fatigue.

WARNING
Lavender essential oil is perfectly safe for home use.

LEMON • CITRUS LIMON

EXTRACTION
Oil is extracted from the fresh rind of the fruit from the citrus tree. It is grown commercially in Spain, Florida, Portugal, Italy, Israel and California.

HERBAL TRADITION
Lemon was used by the ancient Romans for stomach upsets and to sweeten the breath, by the British Navy to prevent scurvy, and it is now used for almost everything, from the cure for sore throats and colds to the slice with ice in a glass of fizzy water.

PROPERTIES
The essential oil has a tangy, fresh, citrus smell and is stimulating, invigorating, astringent, deodorising, diuretic and antiseptic.

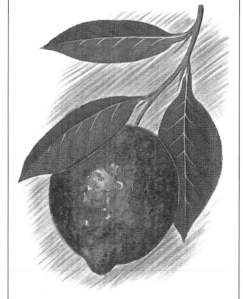

ACTIONS
In aromatherapy it is useful for clearing the head, whether you have a cold or are mentally exhausted, for energising an aching body, for boosting circulation, treating cellulite or warming hands and feet.

HOME USE
Massage, baths, inhalation, poultice. A few drops in a hot bath on a cold night will boost your circulation. Inhale it from a tissue to counter tiredness or to relieve the symptoms of a cold. Use it on a cloth to disinfect or deodorise around the house or in a sickroom.

WARNING
Lemon essential oil should be used in moderation as it may irritate skin, especially if it is exposed to sunshine after application. Store in a cool, dark place.

LEMONGRASS • CYMBOPOGON CITRATUS

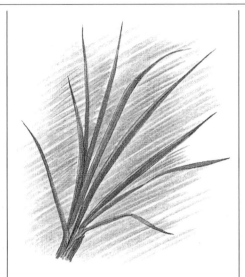

EXTRACTION
Oil is extracted from the fresh or dried wild grass. It is grown commercially in India, Sri Lanka, Indonesia, Africa and the West Indies.

HERBAL TRADITION
Lemongrass is also known as fevergrass as it has been used for centuries to treat fever in India. It has also traditionally been used to cure skin complaints and was burnt to kill germs. It is now mainly used to flavour foods, drinks and toiletries.

PROPERTIES
The essential oil has a warm lemon, grassy smell and is soothing, healing, invigorating, antiseptic, anti-bacterial and deodorising.

ACTIONS
In aromatherapy it is most useful for open pores, boils, athlete's foot, excess perspiration, headaches, poor circulation and as an insect repellent.

HOME USE
Massage, baths, inhalation, poultice, compress. Diluted well and massaged directly onto inflamed skin, armpits, feet and hands, it will boost the circulation, speed healing and deodorise. Apply the oil directly to curtain hems to repel insects, and to shoes or rubbish bins to deodorise. A few drops in a hand or footbath will warm the extremities and reduce sweating.

WARNING
Lemongrass essential oil is perfectly safe for home use as long as it is well diluted.

LIME • CITRUS AURANTIFOLIA

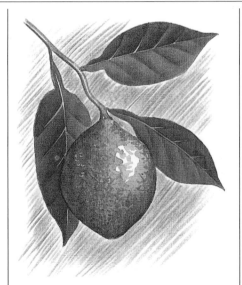

EXTRACTION
Oil is extracted from the peel of the unripe citrus fruit. Today, limes are grown for their oil in Florida, Mexico, Italy and the West Indies.

HERBAL TRADITION
Limes, like lemons, were originally given to British sailors who ate the fruit to reduce the risk of scurvy: hence the nickname, 'limey'. Today it is used as a flavouring in food and drink and a fragrance in cleansers and male toiletries.

PROPERTIES
The essential oil has a sharp, sweet citrus peel smell and is antiseptic, anti-viral, anti-bacterial and is a good warming stimulant and tonic.

ACTIONS
In aromatherapy it is useful for greasy skin, varicose veins, arthritis, rheumatism, poor circulation, cellulite, breathing problems, colds, flu, fever or infection.

HOME USE
Massage, bath, inhalation, poultice. It is good for a leg, anti-cellulite or warming friction massage, or diluted and rubbed into the chest for colds, or as an astringent facial. It makes an excellent warming bath in winter, or a refreshing, energising bath in summer. It can be applied as a poultice for fever or inhaled for any breathing problems or congestion.

WARNING
Lime essential oil should be used in moderation as it may irritate skin, especially if it is exposed to sunshine after application. Store in a cool, dark place.

MANDARIN • CITRUS RETICULATA

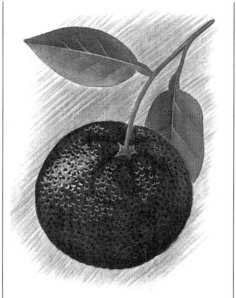

EXTRACTION
Oil is extracted from the peel of the ripe fruit of the citrus tree. It is native to southern China and the Far East but is now grown for oil in Brazil, Mexico, Italy, Florida and the West Indies.

HERBAL TRADITION
Mandarin is named because the fruit was a traditional gift to the Mandarin lords of China for centuries, although the fruit did not reach Europe until the 1880s. Today it is used as to flavour drinks and food, and as a fragrance in perfume and toiletries.

PROPERTIES
The essential oil has a sweet, oranges-and-lemons smell and is a sedative, digestive and has a calming effect.

ACTIONS
In aromatherapy it is used for stretch marks, scars, fluid retention and for stress, irritability, insomnia, restlessness and nervous tension.

HOME USE
Massage, baths, inhalation. It makes a wonderful slimming massage for buttocks, hips and thighs, and will also reduce stretch marks. Put a few drops in a hot bath for a deeply relaxing and uplifting soak, or inhale a few drops from a tissue whenever you feel tense or tired.

WARNING
Mandarin essential oil should be used in moderation as it may irritate skin, especially if it is exposed to sunshine after application. Store in a cool, dark place.

MARIGOLD • CALENDULA OFFICINALIS

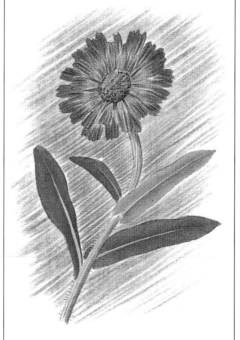

EXTRACTION
Oil is extracted from the flowers of the herb. It is native to the Mediterranean and is grown commercially in Morocco, France, Bulgaria, Hungary and northern Europe.

HERBAL TRADITION
Marigold, otherwise known as calendula, has been used as a folk remedy for centuries, to treat skin problems, strengthen weak eyes and comfort the heart and spirits. Today it is used for nappy rash, varicose veins, dry, cracked or sensitive skin.

PROPERTIES
The essential oil has a musky, woody, slightly unpleasant smell and is a soothing, very therapeutic agent.

ACTIONS
In aromatherapy it is best for healing and soothing burns, cuts, eczema, itchiness, over-dry, inflamed or sensitive skin. It is also excellent for insect bites, rashes or sunburn.

HOME USE
Massage, baths. Although marigold is a excellent healer, the smell can be off-putting, so it is best used in small doses. Add a few drops to a warm bath for skin complaints, or dilute it with a carrier oil and massage in.

WARNING
Calendula essential oil is perfectly safe for home use if well diluted before application.

MARJORAM • ORIGANUM MAJORANA

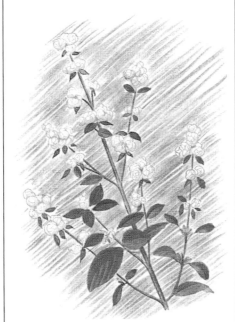

EXTRACTION
Oil is extracted from the dried flowering heads of the shrub. It originated in Asia but is now grown all over Europe and cultivated for oil in Tunisia, Morocco, Germany, Hungary and Egypt.

HERBAL TRADITION
Marjoram was sacred in India and Egypt, and for the Greeks it was a symbol of enduring love. All ancient civilisations used it for digestive, nervous and respiratory complaints.

PROPERTIES
The essential oil has a spicy, peppery, camphor-and-thyme smell and is relaxing, soothing, warming and fortifying.

ACTIONS
In aromatherapy it is useful for headaches, insomnia, tension, bruises, aches, pains, sprains, chilblains, lumbago, bronchitis, coughs and colds.

HOME USE
Massage, baths, inhalation. A few drops in a hot bath boost the circulation and lift the spirits, as well as soothing any aches or muscular pains. For massage, it is particularly good for a stiff neck, headache, migraine, aching joints, muscular pain or after excessive exercise. Inhale it with steam to relieve a chesty cough or congestion.

WARNING
Marjoram is perfectly safe for home use as long as it is well diluted before application. Do not use it during pregnancy.

MIMOSA • ACACIA DEALBATA

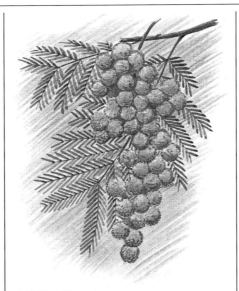

EXTRACTION
Oil is extracted from the bright, pom-pom-like flowers and twig ends of the tree. It is native to Australia but now grows in Europe and is cultivated in France and Italy.

HERBAL TRADITION
The Australian Aborigine has used the 'wattle' tree medicinally for centuries, particularly to treat tummy upsets, diarrhoea, cuts and infected wounds. Today the bark, which is rich in tannins, is used by the leather industry.

PROPERTIES
The essential oil has a sweet, honey-like, green, floral smell and is relaxing, soothing, calming, antiseptic and astringent.

ACTIONS
In aromatherapy it is useful for general skin care and invaluable for its cheering effect, to treat depression, melancholy, emotional upset, over-sensitivity or any kind of nervous tension.

HOME USE
Massage, baths, inhalation. Added to a warm bath, it is an uplifting soak that will soothe your spirits as much as your skin. It makes a lovely scalp, neck or face massage. And a few drops added to a bowl of hot water on a radiator will put everyone who enters into a happier mood.

WARNING
Mimosa essential oil is perfectly safe for home use as long as it is well diluted before application.

MYRRH • COMMIPHORA MYRRHA

EXTRACTION
Oil is extracted from resin collected from the stem and shoots of the tree. It grows in north Africa, northern India and the Middle East.

HERBAL TRADITION
Myrrh, one of three gifts given to the infant Jesus, was much prized by the ancient civilisations. It was used for incense, embalming, perfume, religious ceremonies, and medicinally to treat wounds and chest complaints.

PROPERTIES
The essential oil has a rich, spicy, camphorish smell. It is warming, relaxing, healing, anti-inflammatory, antiseptic, astringent and a good expectorant.

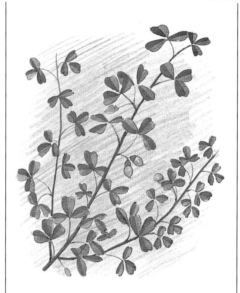

ACTIONS
In aromatherapy it is excellent for healing skin, for eczema, mature complexions, poor circulation, arthritis and any chest or nasal congestion.

HOME USE
Massage, baths, inhalation. Myrrh is wonderful as a wintery oil since it has such a rich smell and warming effect. A few drops in a bath relieves stress. Or use it for an anti-wrinkle, facial massage, a soothing hand massage, a warming foot massage or for any dry skin. Inhaled from a tissue or with steam it relieves a chesty cough and is a good expectorant.

WARNING
Myrrh essential oil is perfectly safe for home use as long as it is well diluted before application. However it should not be used during pregnancy.

NEROLI • CITRUS AURANTIUM BIGARADIA

EXTRACTION
Oil is extracted from the freshly picked blossoms of the bitter orange tree. It is grown commercially in Italy, France, North Africa and Sicily.

HERBAL TRADITION
Neroli oil was discovered in the late 1600s and it was said to be named after Anne-Marie, Princess of Neroli, in Italy. The Roman god Jupiter gave an orange to his sister Juno when he married her, and brides have carried the blossom to calm nerves ever since.

PROPERTIES
The essential oil has a smell that is true to nature, of wonderful, bitter-orangey blossom. It is a hypnotic sedative, calming, relaxing and anti-depressant.

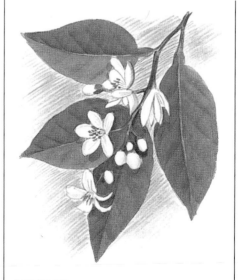

ACTIONS
In aromatherapy it is excellent for any kind of stress or tension, over-excitement, anxiety, insomnia or fears, and it is excellent for improving dry or mature complexions.

HOME USE
Massage, baths, inhalation. Since neroli is a natural tranquilliser, use it with other relaxing oils for the sweetest bath imaginable. It is wonderful for any relaxing massage – back, scalp, neck, face, hand or foot – and improves skin texture at the same time. It is an ideal and safe oil to use during pregnancy. And to feel happy in the face of adversity, inhale a few drops from a tissue or scent your entire house with its calm, sensual smell.

WARNING
Neroli essential oil is perfectly safe for home use. All citrus oils need to be stored in a cool, dark place to preserve them and keep them fresh.

ORANGE • CITRUS SINENSIS

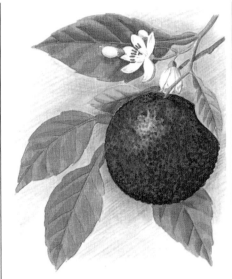

EXTRACTION
Oil is extracted from the fresh fruit peel of the sweet orange tree. The tree grows worldwide, but oil is produced mainly in Italy, France, Spain, Florida, California, Israel and Brazil.

HERBAL TRADITION
Oranges are used extensively in Chinese medicine. The Romans drank orange-flower water after orgies to reduce hangovers. It has been used to boost the immune system and fight colds.

PROPERTIES
The essential oil is almost 90 per cent limonene, which is why it refreshes and stimulates while at the same time leaving you relaxed. It is a good skin rejuvenator.

ACTIONS
In aromatherapy it is excellent for calming children, or anyone who is lethargic or over-tired. Use it for sun exposed skin, wrinkles or a dull, sallow complexion.

HOME USE
Massage, baths, inhalation, poultice, compress. It is useful for massage when you need to relax after a hard day but still need the energy to go out that night, or for any facial massage. It makes an excellent body moisturiser, and, added to the bath, calms fractious children.

WARNING
Orange essential oil should be used in moderation as it may irritate skin, especially if it is exposed to sunshine after application. Store in a cool, dark place.

PATCHOULI • POGOSTEMON CABLIN

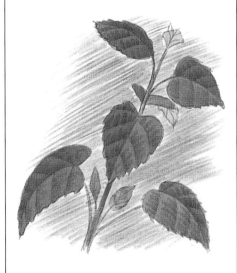

EXTRACTION
Oil is extracted from the dried leaves and shoots of the bushy herb. It is cultivated in India, China, Indonesia, Malaysia and South America.

HERBAL TRADITION
Patchouli has been a much-prized herb in the East since ancient times. It was used to scent linen and clothes. It reached the West in the 19th century when it was used to perfume paisley shawls. It is still used extensively in modern perfumery and was worn alone as the symbol of peace and love by hippies during the 60s.

PROPERTIES
The essential oil has a woody, earthy, sweet smell that is pungent and persistent. It stimulates in small amounts and sedates when used more generously. It is anti-inflammatory and antiseptic.

ACTIONS
In aromatherapy, it is used for tiredness, tension, burns, acne, dandruff, eczema, and oily skin or scalp. It is a heady, sensual oil.

HOME USE
Massage, baths, inhalation, poultice, compress. It makes a relaxing or energising body massage, a therapeutic head and scalp massage and a good oily-skin facial. A few drops in the bath will stimulate if used in moderation, or sedate if used in larger amounts.

WARNING
Patchouli essential oil is perfectly safe for home use as long as it is diluted before application.

PEPPERMINT • MENTHA PIPERITA

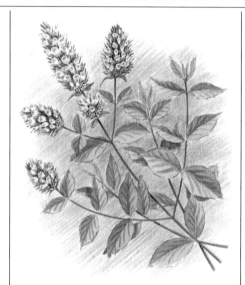

EXTRACTION
Oil is extracted from the fresh or semi-dried leaves and flowers of the herb. The plant is cultivated in Britain, America, Europe and China, but grows worldwide.

HERBAL TRADITION
Mint was prized in Japan and China for centuries and has been found in Egyptian tombs dating back to 1000BC. Traditionally, people drank it as a tea or chewed the leaves to cure 'complaints of the stomach or nerves'.

PROPERTIES
The essential oil is nearly one third menthol, which is why it invigorates, clears the head, stimulates and is soothing, refreshing and cooling.

ACTIONS
In aromatherapy, it is excellent for headaches, mental fatigue, muscular pain, varicose veins, sunburn, insect bites, nausea, indigestion, PMT, or menopausal hot flushes.

HOME USE
Massage, baths, inhalation, compress. A few drops on a tissue can clear your head, whether you're suffering from a cold or mental fatigue, and relieve headaches or any nausea, from travel to morning sickness. Four drops in a basin will refresh tired feet. Use sparingly for massage or in the bath.

WARNING
Mint essential oil is very potent, so never apply undiluted to skin, or just before going to sleep. Always use in moderation.

PETITGRAIN • CITRUS AUANTIUM AMARA

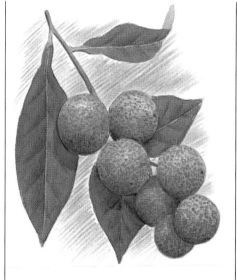

EXTRACTION
Oil is extracted from the leaves and twigs of the bitter orange tree. Today it is grown commercially in France, North Africa and South America.

HERBAL TRADITION
Petitgrain has been used in eau de Cologne for hundreds of years because of its refreshing, stimulating and deodorising effects. Today it is used in perfumery, cosmetics and as a flavouring for drinks.

PROPERTIES
The essential oil has a tangy, sharp, orange smell and combines both relaxing and stimulating properties. It is ideal as a remedy for any form of stress or tiredness.

ACTIONS
In aromatherapy, it is very effective in treating insomnia, fatigue, low energy, backache, muscular tension or any kind of nervousness.

HOME USE
Massage, baths, inhalation. To relax after a hard day or help cure sleeplessness, add the essential oil to a warm bath. For tension, massage into the lower spine, upper back, nape of the neck and temples. And for instant relief from fatigue or nerves, inhale a few drops from a tissue.

WARNING
Petitgrain essential oil is perfectly safe for home use. All citrus oils need to be stored in a cool, dark place to preserve them and keep them fresh.

PINE (LONGLEAF) • PINUS PALUSTRIS

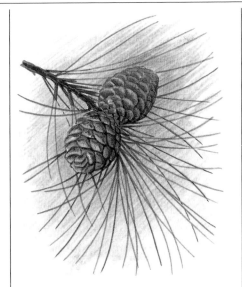

EXTRACTION
Oil is extracted from the needles, cones and twigs of the tree. It is grown commercially in Northern Europe and North America.

HERBAL TRADITION
Pine was used by the ancient Greeks and Romans for respiratory problems and muscular aches, as it still is in saunas throughout Scandinavia. The needles were burnt to drive away insects, infections and clean rooms of germs.

PROPERTIES
The essential oil has a very strong, balsamic, camphor smell similar to crushed pine needles and is both stimulating and antiseptic.

ACTIONS
In aromatherapy, it is a strong germ-killer and tonic, excellent for any viral infections such as coughs, colds and flu, and for muscular aches, rheumatism or arthritis.

HOME USE
Massage, baths, inhalation, poultice. For a cough or blocked nose, massage into the chest. Rub into aching joints. In the bath it improves circulation and relieves muscular pain. Used undiluted on a damp cloth, it makes an effective household disinfectant for the bathroom or to deodorise shoes.

WARNING
ine essential oil is perfectly safe for home use as long as it is well diluted before application.

ROSE • ROSA DAMASCENEA, ROSA CENTIFOLIA

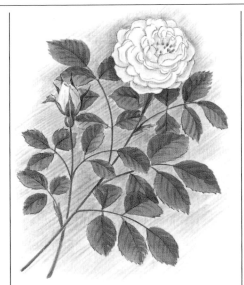

EXTRACTION
Oil is extracted from the freshly picked petals of the rose blossom. It is cultivated mainly in France, Morocco, Bulgaria, China and India, but grows worldwide.

HERBAL TRADITION
Rose was loved by the gods, written about by poets, given to loved ones and, today, still titillates the most jaded nose. The Romans said rosewater banished hangovers and its sensual scent helped orgies continue all night.

PROPERTIES
The essential oil has a smell as sweet as the flower. Both are so well loved that they have an instant uplifting, positive effect.

ACTIONS
In aromatherapy, it is used for stress, depression, headaches, or insomnia. Rose is excellent for the skin, particularly wrinkles, puffiness, broken veins and dryness.

HOME USE
Massage, baths, inhalation. Since the smell gives a feeling of happiness and pleasure, as well as being romantic, it is an excellent oil to scent a room. Use it for facial or full body massages and add ten drops to the bath to relieve a headache or hangover, or to recover from a hard day.

WARNING
Rose essential oil is perfectly safe for home use as long as it is diluted before application.

ROSEMARY • ROSMARINUS OFFICINALIS

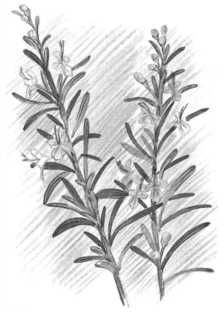

EXTRACTION
Oil is extracted from the flowering tops of the shrubby evergreen bush. It is grown commercially in England, the Mediterranean, California and China.

HERBAL TRADITION
Rosemary has long been valued as a sacred plant. It has been used for magic, medicine and on the menus of most early civilisations. It is burnt to drive away infection, eaten for liver and digestive disorders, and inhaled for respiratory and nervous complaints.

PROPERTIES
The essential oil has a fresh, green, woody, mint smell and is antiseptic, stimulating, astringent, invigorating and cleansing.

ACTIONS
In aromatherapy, it is used for headaches, breathing problems, fluid retention, poor circulation or dandruff.

HOME USE
Massage, baths, inhalation. It is particularly useful as a warming body massage for any muscular aches, or as a head and scalp massage for greasiness, lack of concentration or headaches. Add it to the bath as a pick-me-up for mental or physical tiredness and inhale it for coughs, bronchitis and other breathing problems.

WARNING
Rosemary essential oil is perfectly safe for home use as long as it is well diluted before application. However, do not use it during pregnancy or if you have epilepsy (or if you are giving a massage to someone suffering from the condition).

ROSEWOOD • ANIBA ROSAEODORA

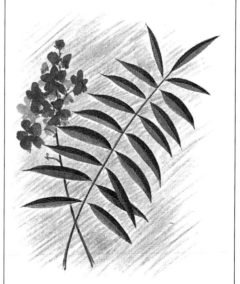

EXTRACTION
Oil is extracted from the wood of the tropical, evergreen tree. It is grown commercially in Brazil and Peru.

HERBAL TRADITION
Rosewood was most valued for the fragrant wood, particularly used for 19th-century English furniture. The Amazon Indians used it medicinally for wounds and skin complaints. Today the wood is used for chopsticks, as the oil in some soaps and toiletries and to flavour food and drinks.

PROPERTIES
The essential oil has a sweet, floral, woody smell and is soothing, healing, deodorising, relaxing, tonic, calming, and gently sensual.

ACTIONS
In aromatherapy it is most useful for any skin problems, from acne, scars and wrinkles to dull, dry complexions. It is an intimate, deeply relaxing oil.

HOME USE
Massage, baths, inhalation. From a full body massage, to a facial, it benefits both skin and mood in one clean sweep. Added to a bath it helps round out other oils and is liked by both men and women equally. It also makes an excellent, intimate, relaxing room scent.

WARNING
Rosewood essential oil is perfectly safe for home use as long as it is diluted before application.

SAGE (CLARY) • CALIVA SCLAREA

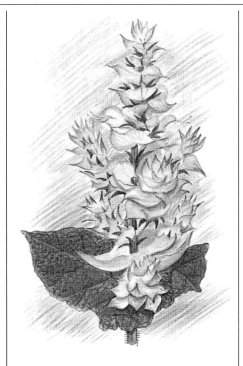

EXTRACTION
Oil is extracted from the flowering tops and leaves of the perennial herb. It is grown for oil in Morocco, England, France and throughout the Mediterranean.

HERBAL TRADITION
Clary sage was once one of the most valued herbs, used for stomach disorders, infertility and all nervous problems. In Latin 'clary' means clear eye; the herb was so named because it made a soothing, healing eye lotion.

PROPERTIES
The essential oil has a green, balsamic, aromatic smell and is mildly antiseptic, an uplifting tonic, warming and relaxing.

ACTIONS
In aromatherapy, it is useful for PMT and menstrual cramps, for depression, fatigue, stress, headaches and skin inflammations or irritations.

HOME USE
Massage, baths. A few drops in the bath soothe backache, pains and sprains, cramps, bad moods, itchy skin and will leave you energised. It is good for face, neck and scalp massages to help banish headaches and tension.

WARNING
Clary sage is perfectly safe for home use as long as it is well diluted before application. However, do not use it during pregnancy.

SANDALWOOD • SANTALUM ALBUM

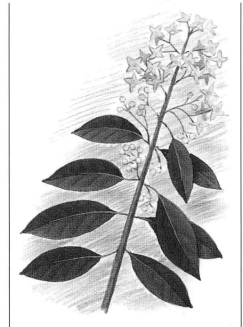

EXTRACTION
Oil is extracted from the roots and heart wood of the tree. Most oil comes from India, but it is also cultivated in Malaysia, Sri Lanka and Indonesia.

HERBAL TRADITION
Sandalwood has long been a favourite perfume ingredient, and the ancient Egyptians, Chinese and Indians used it for incense and embalming. Medicinally, it has been used to cure skin inflammations and to help discharge mucus.

PROPERTIES
The essential oil has a deep fruity-sweet woody smell and is antiseptic, astringent, relaxing, sedative and regarded as an aphrodisiac.

ACTIONS
In aromatherapy, it is used for insomnia, tension, stress, depression, loss of libido, emotional problems and cracked or chapped skin. It is also a good expectorant for coughs or colds.

HOME USE
Massage, baths, inhalation, compress. A few drops in a hot bath make one of the most soothing, sensual soaks that will cleanse both mind and body. It makes the most relaxing body massage and is particularly good for any patches of rough, dry skin. Inhaled with steam or as a poultice it clears any congestion.

WARNING
Sandalwood essential oil is perfectly safe for home use as long as it is diluted before application.

SPRUCE • *TSUGA CANADENSIS*

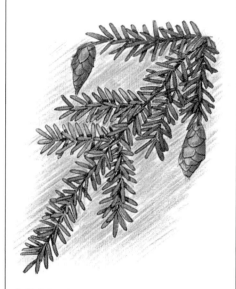

EXTRACTION
Oil is extracted from the needles and twigs of the large evergreen tree. It is native to the west coast of North America and is grown there extensively for oil.

HERBAL TRADITION
The hemlock spruce was used medicinally by the American Indians. They made a tisane from the bark and burned the branches to cure fever and infection. Today a tannin extract from the bark is used in the leather industry.

PROPERTIES
The essential oil has a clean, fresh, sweet balsamic smell and is antiseptic, warming, astringent, soothing, calming and relaxing.

ACTIONS
In aromatherapy it is used for sprains, stiffness and pain, poor circulation, cellulite, rheumatism and coughs or colds, and to reduce anxiety and stress.

HOME USE
Massage, baths, inhalation, poultice. Apply on a hot poultice or dilute and use as a linament to rub into stiff, aching or over-exercised muscles. It makes a warming winter massage for feet and legs, to boost the circulation, tone and reduce cellulite. In the bath it has a soothing, sedative effect and is pleasantly relaxing. Inhaled with steam, it helps you sleep through the congestion that comes with a bad cold.

WARNING
Spruce essential oil is perfectly safe for home use as long as it is well diluted before application.

TARRAGON • *ARTEMISIA DRACUNCULUS*

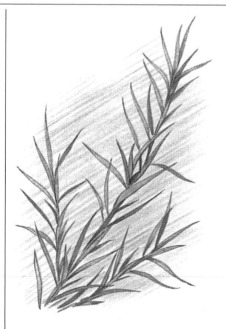

EXTRACTION
Oil is extracted from the leaves of the bushy perennial plant. It is widely grown, but most oil comes from France, Holland and America.

HERBAL TRADITION
Tarragon was used in the Middle East for flatulence. When the Crusaders brought it to Europe it was said to protect against the bites of mad dogs, dragons and other beasts! Today it is used as a flavouring for food and condiments.

PROPERTIES
The essential oil has an anise or fennel smell with a spicy, green edge. It is calming, antispasmodic, antiseptic, digestive and slightly diuretic.

ACTIONS
In aromatherapy, it is useful for any stomach complaints, from nervous butterflies or knots in the tummy, to indigestion, flatulence, PMT, cramps or constipation.

HOME USE
Massage, poultice, compress. For any stomach problems, massage the well-diluted essential oil in slow, circular, palm-stroke movements, clockwise around the abdomen. For cramps, wind or indigestion, apply a hot poultice steeped in the oil. It is not recommended for the bath.

WARNING
Tarragon essential oil is perfectly safe for home use if well diluted and used in moderation. However, do not use it during pregnancy.

TEA-TREE • MELALEUCA ALTERNIFOLIA

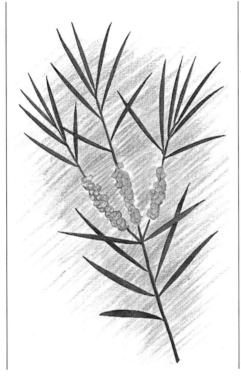

EXTRACTION
Oil is extracted from the leaves and twigs of the shrub. Native to Australia, all the oil is produced there.

HERBAL TRADITION
Tea-tree was named by Captain Cook's crew, who brewed the small, dark leaves and drank it as a tea substitute. Its astounding healing properties were used by the Aborigines. During World War II medics recognised its powerful germicidal and antiseptic effects.

PROPERTIES
The essential oil has a spicy, hot, nutmeg-like, medicinal smell and is a powerful, non-irritating antiseptic that kills bacteria, fungi and virus 12 times as effectively as carbolic.

ACTIONS
In aromatherapy, it is used for cuts, burns, acne, stings, blisters, herpes and nappy rash. It is very effective in treating yeast and fungal infections.

HOME USE
Massage, baths, inhalation, poultice. Diluted one part essential oil to nine parts carrier oil, it makes an instant home first-aid kit. Apply to cuts, burns, spots, stings and other irritations. Add it to the bath or use as a douche for viral or fungal infections.

WARNING
Warning: Tea-tree essential oil is perfectly safe for home use as long as it is diluted before application.

THYME (WHITE) • THYMUS VULGARIS

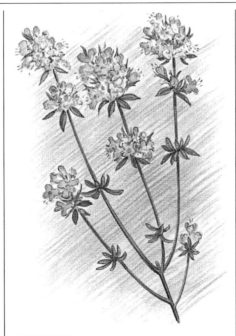

EXTRACTION
Oil is extracted from the fresh or dried leaves and flowering tops of the perennial herbaceous plant. It is grown for oil in Spain, Morocco, France, Algeria, Israel and Greece.

HERBAL TRADITION
The ancient Egyptians used thyme for embalming, the Greeks and Romans for medicinal purposes. It is said to have been added to the hay in baby Jesus' crib and to be sewn into knight's clothing to keep them brave in battle.

PROPERTIES
The essential oil contains thymol (a powerful antiseptic) and has a tangy, herby smell. It is a good stimulant, expectorant, and insect repellent.

ACTIONS
In aromatherapy, it is most useful for tension, fatigue, anxiety, headaches, skin irritations, coughs, colds and rheumatic aches and pains. It is disliked by most flying insects.

HOME USE
Massage, baths, inhalation. Mixed with other anti-stress oils, it makes an invigorating bath. It is good to massage in for aching muscles, headaches and rheumatic pain. Inhaled with steam, it is excellent for breathing problems.

WARNING
White thyme is perfectly safe for home use if well diluted before application and used in moderation. However, do not use during pregnancy. Red thyme is toxic and should not be used at all.

VALERIAN • VALERIANA FAURIEI

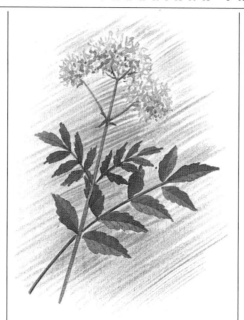

EXTRACTION
Oil is extracted from the roots of the perennial herb. It is grown for the oil in England, Belgium, France and Holland.

HERBAL TRADITION
Valerian has been valued as a healing cure-all herb throughout Europe since medieval times. It was tucked inside pillows to induce sleep and calm women who took to their beds complaining of nerves, and placed in sickrooms to speed recovery, lift spirits and relieve pain.

PROPERTIES
The essential oil has a warm, mossy, musky woody smell and is hypnotic, calming, soothing and sedative.

ACTIONS
In aromatherapy, it is excellent for treating sleeplessness, tension, nerves, melancholy, moodiness and irritability.

HOME USE
Massage, baths, inhalation. A few drops on a tissue placed by a pillow at night will help sedate children or adults. In a warm bath, it is calming and hypnotic. And when used for a slow, soothing massage it overcomes insomnia, irritation and bad moods.

WARNING
Valerian essential oil is perfectly safe for home use as long as it is well diluted before application and used in moderation.

VIOLET • VIOLA ODORATA

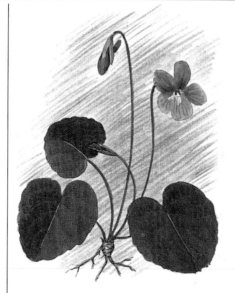

EXTRACTION
Oil is extracted from the fresh leaves and flowers of the perennial plant. It is grown for oil in southern France, Italy and China.

HERBAL TRADITION
The leaf and flowers, with their sweet smell, have long been valued medicinally. The plant was used as a skin-soother and complexion-brightener. A tisane was drunk to relieve nerves and headaches.

PROPERTIES
The essential oil has a delicate floral and potent green-leaf combination and it is anti-inflammatory, astringent, antiseptic, circulation boosting, soothing, light and refreshing.

ACTIONS
In aromatherapy, it is useful for any skin irritation or inflammation, particularly thread veins, open pores, acne, blackheads, eczema, spots and rashes. It also relieves headaches, dizziness, emotional turmoil, clears the head and improves concentration.

HOME USE
Massage, baths, inhalation. Use it for any beautifying facial massage, and once diluted, smooth it onto skin morning and night to rejuvenate any complexion. A few drops in the bath will turn you into a clear-headed quick thinker after a day of concentration. It will also relieve headaches and emotional upset.

WARNING
Violet essential oil is perfectly safe for home use as long as it is diluted before application.

YARROW • ACHILLEA MILLEFOLIUM

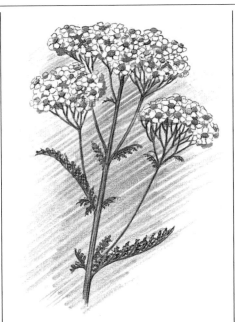

EXTRACTION
Oil is extracted from the leaves and flowers of the dried herb. It is grown commercially in America, Africa, France and Germany.

HERBAL TRADITION
Yarrow is a traditional cure-all used to treat infections, fevers and digestive problems. The Greek warrior Achilles is reputed to have used it to heal battle wounds, until Paris shot him in his one weak spot, his heel. Today it is used to give the bitter taste to vermouths.

PROPERTIES
The essential oil has a fresh, mossy, camphor smell and is anti-inflammatory, antiseptic, astringent, sedative and deeply relaxing.

ACTIONS
In aromatherapy, it is useful for calming nerves, lowering blood pressure, treating insomnia and other stress-related problems. It is also excellent for rashes, scars, acne, oiliness, and promoting healthy hair.

HOME USE
Massage, baths, inhalation. Mixed with other relaxing oils it makes a good massage to relieve sleeplessness. Inhaled from a tissue or as a room scent it helps reduce hypertension and calm nerves. A few drops in a bath soothes skin, or use it for a toning treatment facial.

WARNING
Yarrow essential oil is perfectly safe for home use as long as it is well diluted before application. However, do not use it during pregnancy.

YLANG-YLANG • CANANGA ODORATA

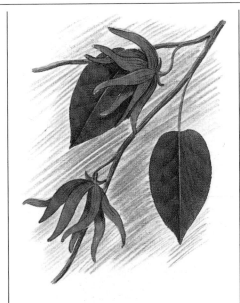

EXTRACTION
Oil is extracted from the freshly picked flower of the tropical tree. It is grown commercially in Madagascar, the Philippines and Reunion Island.

HERBAL TRADITION
Ylang-ylang was used by the islanders of tropical Asia to treat insect bites, inflamed skin, protect their hair and ward off fever or infection. It was first used commercially by the Victorians in Macassar hair oil, an early conditioner and growth-stimulator. Since the flower has so sensual a fragrance, it has always been used to symbolise love.

PROPERTIES
The essential oil has a sweet, potent floral smell, reminiscent of hyacinth or narcissus. It is aromatic, hypnotic, relaxing and effects the mind and emotions more than the body. It also is rejuvenating for skin and hair.

ACTIONS
In aromatherapy, it is useful for calming tension, lifting negative moods and increasing sensuality.

HOME USE
Massage, baths, inhalation. It is such a potent, sweet smell that it is best used sparingly. A few drops in any massage or bath will soothe away stress, improve your mood and stimulate the senses. It is one of the best oils for calming and relaxing without sedating.

WARNING
Ylang-ylang essential oil is perfectly safe for home use as long as it is well diluted before application and used in moderation.

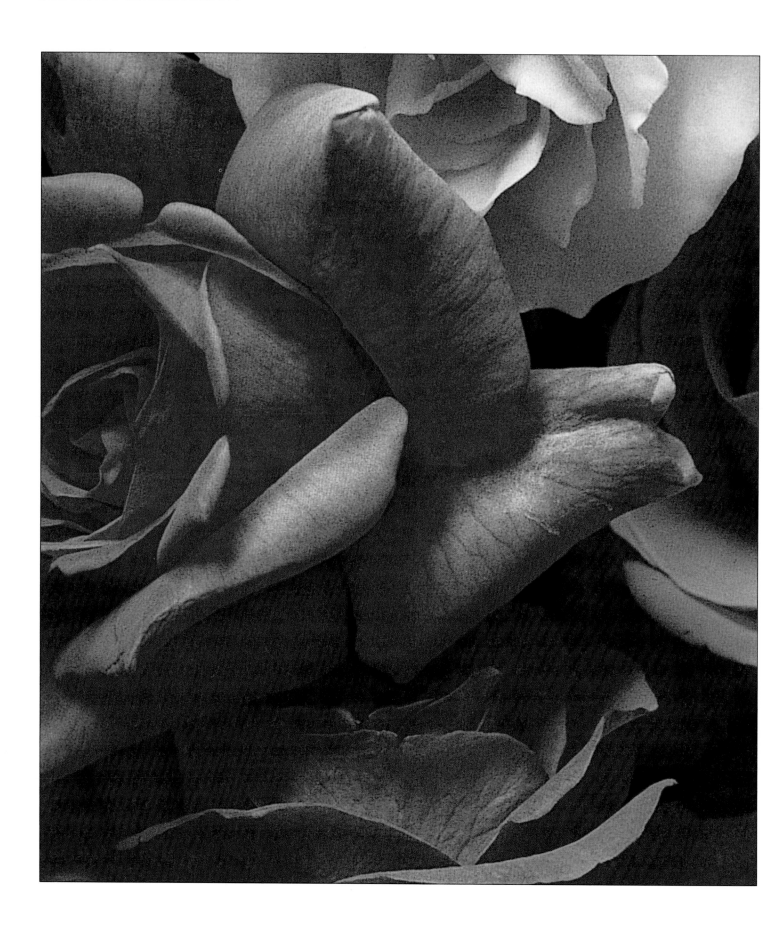

The Best Oils to Buy

The main rule when it comes to buying essential oils is to be led by your nose. Since our sense of smell is so closely linked to our memories and feelings about each aroma, it is a very personal thing. Your best friend might love eucalyptus because it reminds her of a holiday in Australia, while all it does for you is fill you with the fear you had as a child in hospital with pneumonia.

On your first buying trip, do not try to sniff every oil in the shop. There are so many, you'll only end up being confused. The human nose tires quickly and switches off if it is bombarded with different aromas, so take a list of the ten oils you are most interested in from a therapeutic point of view and start by sniffing those.

Good Mixers

In general, the most useful oils are those that mix well with as many other oils as possible. They also need to have the broadest range of therapeutic uses combined with the most pleasant aromas possible. Here is an ideal small collection:

To start with: *jasmine • lavender • neroli • peppermint • rose • sandalwood*
Useful extras: *chamomile • eucalyptus • geranium • lemon • patchouli • ylang-ylang*

The Fragrance Families

Another way to reduce the number of essential oils you choose from initially is to establish which fragrance categories you instinctively prefer. To find out, turn to the sniff-tests on page 14. The five main groups are green, spicy, floral, citrus and balsamic/woody. Nobody likes all of them equally. Once you know your preference, concentrate on the essential oils that fall into those categories (see below) and make those among the first you buy for your collection.

Green	Spicy	Floral	Citrus	Woody/Balsamic
basil	camphor	geranium	bergamot	ambrette
chamomile	fennel	jasmine	citronella	angelica
clary sage	ginger	lavender	lemon	bay
eucalyptus	juniper	mimosa	lemongrass	birch
galbanum	laurel	neroli	lime	cedarwood
peppermint	marjoram	rose	mandarin	frankincense
pine	myrrh	rosewood	orange	marigold
rosemary	tarragon	violet	petitgrain	patchouli
spruce	tea-tree	ylang-ylang		sandalwood
thyme				valerian
				yarrow

MIXING ESSENTIAL OILS

	Ambrete Seed	Angelica	Basil	Bay	Bergamot	Birch (White)	Camphor (White)	Cedarwood (Atlas)	Chamomile (German)	Citronella	Cypress	Eucalyptus	Fennel	Frankincense	Galbanum	Geranium	Ginger	Jasmine	Juniper	Laurel	Lavender	Lemon	Lemongrass	Lime
Ambrete Seed		■		■					■		■					■	■		■		■	■		■
Angelica	■							■	■		■			■	■						■			
Basil				■				■			■			■		■	■			■	■	■	■	■
Bay			■		■	■	■	■			■					■					■	■		
Bergamot	■		■	■				■	■	■		■		■		■	■	■			■	■		■
Birch (White)				■						■		■			■						■			
Camphor (White)				■				■					■			■			■					■
Cedarwood (Atlas)			■	■		■		■		■	■	■		■		■		■	■		■	■		■
Chamomile (German)		■		■				■			■		■			■		■			■			
Citronella	■	■	■		■		■				■				■		■				■	■	■	■
Cypress		■	■	■	■	■		■	■			■		■		■					■	■		
Eucalyptus	■	■	■	■				■	■		■			■		■								
Fennel			■	■	■		■	■		■	■			■		■					■			
Frankincense		■			■	■	■	■		■	■	■	■			■					■	■	■	■
Galbanum		■		■				■						■							■			
Geranium	■	■	■	■	■							■						■	■		■	■		■
Ginger	■			■	■				■							■		■	■					
Jasmine			■		■									■		■					■	■	■	
Juniper	■										■									■	■			
Laurel				■					■	■						■		■			■			
Lavender	■	■			■		■	■			■			■		■		■				■	■	■
Lemon	■			■	■			■						■		■			■	■				■
Lemongrass		■			■				■					■		■		■			■			
Lime	■		■		■	■	■		■	■				■							■	■		
Mandarin	■								■						■	■	■				■			
Marigold (Calendula)								■	■										■		■	■		■
Marjoram		■		■					■	■		■			■	■			■		■	■	■	
Mimosa		■		■					■					■	■	■		■			■			
Myrrh					■						■			■					■		■	■		
Neroli		■		■			■	■	■					■	■	■	■				■	■		
Orange	■			■			■							■	■	■	■				■	■	■	■
Patchouli			■					■	■	■				■		■	■	■			■			
Peppermint	■		■	■		■	■			■	■				■						■			
Petitgrain	■		■	■																				
Pine	■		■			■	■	■	■		■	■		■						■	■			
Rose		■			■				■	■		■		■	■	■					■			
Rosemary	■		■	■	■		■	■	■	■		■		■	■						■	■		
Rosewood		■		■											■	■		■			■			
Sage (Clary)		■						■													■		■	■
Sandalwood			■	■					■		■	■		■		■		■			■			
Spruce	■	■								■											■			
Tarragon			■		■	■																■		
Tea Tree			■		■					■				■							■	■		
Thyme (White)	■		■		■	■		■		■											■	■		
Valerian					■			■								■					■			
Violet		■						■						■	■						■		■	■
Yarrow								■					■	■	■			■			■			
Ylang-Ylang		■		■									■		■	■	■	■	■		■	■		

This table shows essential oil blending compatibilities. Column headers (left to right): Mandarin, Marigold (Calendula), Marjoram, Mimosa, Myrrh, Neroli, Orange, Patchouli, Peppermint, Petitgrain, Pine, Rose, Rosemary, Rosewood, Sage (Clary), Sandalwood, Spruce, Tarragon, Tea Tree, Thyme (White), Valerian, Violet, Yarrow, Ylang-Ylang.

Oil	Mand	Mari	Marj	Mimo	Myrr	Nero	Oran	Patc	Pepp	Peti	Pine	Rose	Rsmy	Rswd	Sage	Sand	Spru	Tarr	TeaT	Thym	Vale	Viol	Yarr	Ylan
Ambrete Seed	■						■	■	■	■		■				■			■					
Angelica			■		■					■			■								■			
Basil		■						■	■	■		■		■		■	■		■					■
Bay										■				■										
Bergamot		■	■		■	■	■	■	■	■	■	■	■	■			■	■						■
Birch (White)										■						■			■					
Camphor (White)				■				■		■		■				■	■							
Cedarwood (Atlas)			■	■			■			■		■		■						■				
Chamomile (German)	■		■	■		■		■				■	■			■	■		■	■			■	
Citronella		■			■			■				■									■			
Cypress		■		■						■	■	■		■	■									
Eucalyptus		■						■	■	■		■		■			■		■	■				
Fennel								■			■	■				■				■				
Frankincense	■			■	■	■				■	■	■	■			■						■	■	
Galbanum	■			■	■									■								■	■	
Geranium	■		■	■	■	■	■	■			■	■	■	■		■		■		■	■	■	■	■
Ginger			■					■			■	■		■	■	■							■	
Jasmine			■					■			■		■	■	■	■								■
Juniper		■						■	■		■	■										■	■	■
Laurel		■							■			■												
Lavender	■	■		■	■	■	■									■		■	■	■			■	
Lemon	■	■			■	■	■	■								■			■	■			■	
Lemongrass		■						■				■		■			■			■				
Lime		■								■		■								■				
Mandarin			■	■	■	■	■			■		■	■		■					■		■	■	
Marigold (Calendula)												■	■	■						■		■		
Marjoram				■							■	■	■	■	■	■						■		■
Mimosa	■			■	■	■	■	■			■	■	■							■				■
Myrrh			■	■	■					■				■	■	■			■		■			
Neroli	■		■	■	■		■				■	■	■	■						■		■		■
Orange	■			■		■		■		■	■	■	■	■	■					■		■		
Patchouli	■			■	■	■				■	■	■				■								■
Peppermint				■	■				■		■	■												
Petitgrain	■					■						■				■						■	■	
Pine						■	■					■				■	■		■					
Rose	■		■	■	■		■						■	■		■				■		■	■	
Rosemary	■	■	■	■		■	■	■		■	■		■		■	■			■					
Rosewood		■				■	■			■	■			■										■
Sage (Clary)	■		■				■		■		■	■				■						■		■
Sandalwood		■	■	■		■	■	■	■		■	■	■		■		■							■
Spruce		■		■						■		■							■					
Tarragon																								
Tea Tree										■					■									
Thyme (White)												■		■		■								
Valerian				■	■	■	■																	■
Violet	■	■		■																		■		
Yarrow	■	■		■			■		■			■		■						■				
Ylang-Ylang	■		■	■		■		■		■	■	■		■	■	■				■	■			

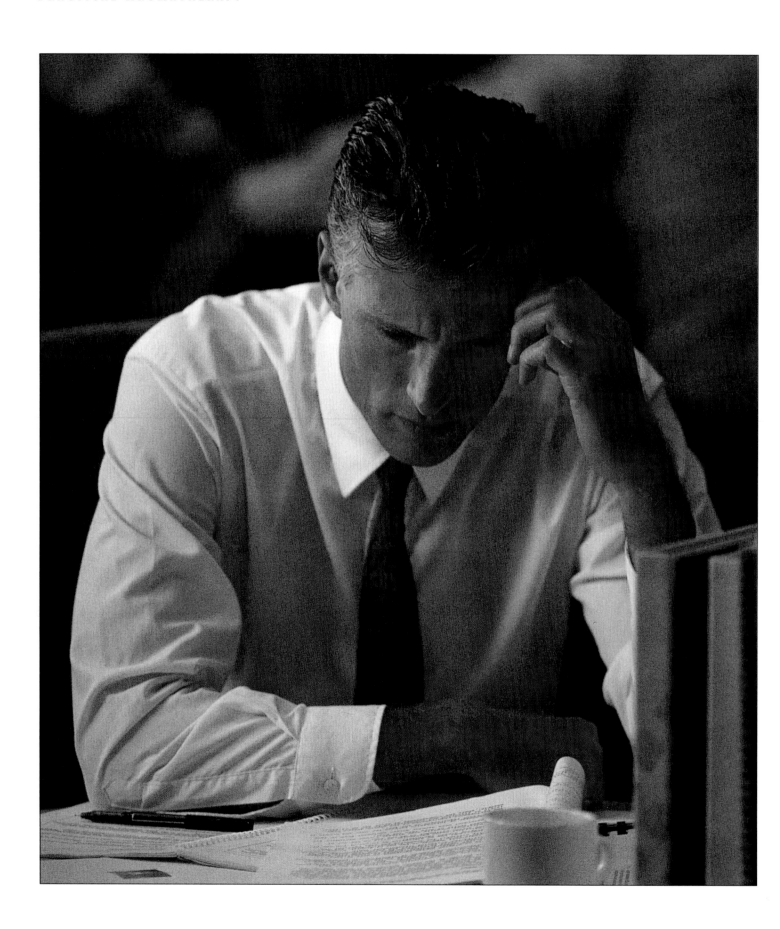

ESSENTIAL OILS FOR COMMON PROBLEMS

Essential oils can be broadly grouped in three categories, according to their general effects. There are those oils that are relaxing and calming, those that are stimulating, and those with a therapeutic effect.

The chart on page 50 gives you a quick guide to which herbs fall into each of the three categories. Should you want an essential oil that will have a relaxing effect, at the same time dealing with a backache, the chart on page 50 will lead you to oils such as ambrette seed, juniper, laurel and lavender.

If you are looking for a treatment for a particular condition, you will find it quickest to turn directly to the relevant entry in the alphabetical listing of common problems, which begins on page 52. This gives you more information on specific ailments or conditions that you can treat using aromatherapy.

For instance, should you want to know more about treating burns, you could turn to the entry on page 54. This gives you some information about the nature of burns, and explains how essential oils can be used to treat them. Each entry includes a list of the best oils for treating that condition. This highlights the general effects of each oil (whether it is relaxing, stimulating or healing), and points out any special features of the oils. In the entry on burns, you will discover that burns can be treated with lavender and tea-tree oils, both of which can be applied undiluted.

For specific information on diluting, combining and mixing the different essential oils, turn to the next chapter, How to Use Essential Oils, which starts on page 65. Be sure to check these guidelines before launching into your treatment: it is very important that essential oils are used in the right way, as some can be toxic if they are misused.

(Left) Use essential oils as a positive way to relieve stress.

USING ESSENTIAL OILS (Index of Common Problems)

MAIN PROPERTIES OF OILS

Ⓡ RELAXING, CALMING

Ⓣ THERAPEUTIC

Ⓢ STIMULATING, UPLIFTING

Problem	Ⓢ Ⓡ Ambrette Seed	Ⓡ Ⓣ Angelica	Ⓢ Ⓣ Basil	Ⓢ Bay	Ⓢ Ⓡ Bergamot	Ⓣ Birch (White)	Ⓢ Camphor (White)	Ⓡ Cedarwood (Atlas)	Ⓡ Ⓣ Chamomile (German)	Ⓣ Citronella	Ⓣ Ⓡ Cypress	Ⓢ Eucalyptus	Ⓡ Fennel	Ⓡ Frankincense	Ⓡ Ⓢ Galbanum	Ⓣ Geranium	Ⓡ Ginger	Ⓣ Ⓡ Jasmine	Ⓣ Ⓡ Juniper	Ⓡ Ⓢ Laurel	Ⓢ Ⓣ Lavender	Ⓢ Lemon	Ⓢ Lemongrass	Ⓢ Lime
ACNE				■			■	■						■				■			■	■	■	
ANXIETY	■		■										■	■		■					■			
ARTHRITIS	■						■		■	■						■		■			■	■		■
ATHLETE'S FOOT					■									■							■		■	
BACKACHE	■		■		■		■										■	■	■					
BITES AND STINGS			■						■	■											■			
BREATHING PROBLEMS		■						■				■												
BRUISES							■			■				■							■			
BUNIONS										■											■			
BURNS							■							■							■			
CELLULITE			■				■		■		■			■				■			■	■		■
CHICKEN POX				■				■		■											■			
CHILBLAINS								■	■							■		■			■	■		
CIRCULATION, POOR		■					■		■							■		■			■	■	■	■
COLDS		■	■		■					■									■		■	■	■	■
COUGHS		■					■		■	■		■				■					■			
CRAMPS							■			■								■	■					
CUTS AND ABRASIONS				■				■	■					■							■			
DANDRUFF			■				■							■				■			■	■		
DEPRESSION			■										■	■		■		■			■			
DERMATITIS/ECZEMA/PSORIASIS			■	■				■		■				■							■			
FATIGUE	■		■	■								■		■	■	■	■				■		■	
FLUID RETENTION					■				■		■			■			■							
HAIR				■	■		■	■	■					■							■	■		
HANGOVER														■							■	■		
HEADACHES	■						■			■		■									■	■		
HERPES					■			■			■										■	■		
HOUSEHOLD CLEANSERS				■				■	■		■				■						■	■	■	■
INDIGESTION	■	■											■								■			
INFLUENZA											■								■					■
INSECT REPELLANT						■				■												■		
INSOMNIA			■						■		■					■		■			■			
JETLAG											■					■					■			
MEASLES					■			■		■											■			
MENOPAUSE								■		■						■					■			
NAUSEA																	■					■		
PERSPIRATION					■					■											■	■		
P.M.T.					■			■				■				■		■	■		■			
RHEUMATISM		■				■		■		■	■					■					■			■
SEXUAL PROBLEMS																■	■	■						
SKIN					■			■				■		■		■		■			■	■		■
STRESS			■		■			■						■		■								
SUNBURN								■						■							■			
THRUSH/CANDIDA/FUNGAL PROBLEMS																		■			■			
TRAVEL SICKNESS					■												■					■		

50

	(R) Mandarin	(T) Marigold (Calendula)	(T)(R) Marjoram	(R) Mimosa	(R)(S) Myrrh	(R) Neroli	(R)(S) Orange	(S)(R) Patchouli	(S)(T) Peppermint	(R)(S) Petitgrain	(S) Pine	(R) Rose	(S)(T) Rosemary	(R) Rosewood	(S)(R) Sage (Clary)	(R) Sandalwood	(S)(R) Spruce	(T) Tarragon	(T)(S) Tea Tree	(T)(S) Thyme (White)	(R)(T) Valerian	(S) Violet	(R) Yarrow	(R) Ylang-Ylang
ACNE					■			■				■	■			■				■			■	
ANXIETY	■		■		■		■		■			■	■	■	■				■	■				■
ARTHRITIS		■		■				■		■		■			■									
ATHLETE'S FOOT																			■					
BACKACHE		■						■	■		■		■		■		■							
BITES AND STINGS		■					■										■							
BREATHING PROBLEMS		■		■				■		■	■			■			■							
BRUISES		■	■										■											
BUNIONS								■									■							
BURNS		■					■				■						■							
CELLULITE							■					■		■		■								
CHICKEN POX																	■							
CHILBLAINS		■									■				■	■								
CIRCULATION, POOR		■		■			■	■		■		■		■		■								■
COLDS				■			■		■					■			■	■						
COUGHS				■			■		■		■				■	■		■						
CRAMPS	■		■			■						■						■						■
CUTS AND ABRASIONS		■														■								
DANDRUFF						■					■			■		■								
DEPRESSION			■	■	■					■		■	■	■						■			■	
DERMATITIS/ECZEMA/PSORIASIS		■		■			■			■				■						■				
FATIGUE				■	■	■	■				■		■						■					
FLUID RETENTION	■					■					■				■									
HAIR							■			■						■					■	■		
HANGOVER				■			■		■															
HEADACHES							■		■	■		■						■		■				
HERPES		■					■									■								
HOUSEHOLD CLEANERS							■		■								■	■						
INDIGESTION	■		■				■											■						
INFLUENZA		■			■		■		■		■				■		■	■						
INSECT REPELLANT																		■	■					
INSOMNIA	■		■		■			■		■			■					■			■	■		
JETLAG							■																	
MEASLES																■								
MENOPAUSE							■		■		■		■		■									■
NAUSEA	■						■																	
PERSPIRATION																	■							
P.M.T.							■		■			■	■		■									
RHEUMATISM		■						■		■			■				■							
SEXUAL PROBLEMS			■	■				■		■	■	■	■											■
SKIN	■	■		■	■	■	■	■		■		■	■	■	■			■	■		■	■	■	■
STRESS		■	■	■						■		■	■	■	■					■		■	■	■
SUNBURN				■						■														
THRUSH/CANDIDA/FUNGAL PROBLEMS				■											■				■					
TRAVEL SICKNESS	■								■															

ACNE

(see also SKIN)

Acne and skin eruptions are caused by the over-production of oil in the sebaceous glands. Poor diet, lack of exercise, stress, anxiety and hormonal fluctuations (often brought on by puberty, menstruation or the menopause) all aggravate the condition. Excess sebum will build up in hair follicles and oily areas around the nose and chin. Essential oils are particularly effective on problem skin because not only are they anti-bacterial, antiseptic and healing, but they also soothe the mental stresses which can make acne worse.

Best Oils: bergamot, cedarwood, geranium, juniper, lavender, lemon, rosewood, sandalwood, yarrow, tea-tree (antiseptic, healing, oil regulators); chamomile and petitgrain (for boils or inflammation); patchouli, lemongrass (cleansing).

ALOPECIA

(see HAIR LOSS)

ANXIETY

(see also STRESS)

Anxiety is caused by the everyday stresses and strains, demands, upsets and worries of life. The symptoms range from headaches, nervousness and knotted, tense muscles to insomnia, low resistance and depression. Essential oils help by reducing negative feelings, relaxing the mind and body and soothing both mood and emotions.

Best Oils: ambrette seed, mimosa, lavender, mandarin, neroli, patchouli, sandalwood, spruce, valerian (calming); bergamot, frankincense, rosewood, violet (uplifting, cheering); jasmine, petitgrain, clary sage ylang-ylang (relaxing, uplifting).

ARTHRITIS

Arthritis is an inflammation of the joints. There are two types: rheumatoid arthritis, which affects the surrounding connective tissue, causing pain, swelling and stiffness; and osteo-arthritis, the wearing away of cartilage, resulting in pain, loss of mobility and swelling. Essential oils can help by relaxing muscles, reducing inflammation and soothing pain, but cannot cure either condition.

Best oils: marjoram, ginger, eucalyptus, juniper, peppermint, pine (warming, relaxing); cypress, lime, myrrh, spruce, ambrette seed, lemon, rosemary (anti-inflammatory, healing).

ATHLETE'S FOOT

Athlete's foot is a fungal infection of the feet. Skin between the toes becomes red, itchy and peels. It is very contagious, often caught from wet floors of communal changing-rooms and showers, where the fungus thrives.

Best oils: lavender (antiseptic, healing); tea-tree (anti-fungal), geranium, birch (anti-inflammatory, soothing); lemongrass (deodorising, drying).

BACKACHE

Backache and muscular pain affect almost everyone at some point in their lives. It may be caused by lifting heavy weights, bad posture, too much or too little exercise, a fall, pregnancy, or even a powerful sneeze.

Best Oils: bay, camphor, citronella, eucalyptus, marjoram, pine, spruce (relaxing, warming); ambrette, petitgrain, juniper, rosemary (soothing, stimulating); lavender, clary sage, thyme (relaxes muscles, anti-inflammatory).

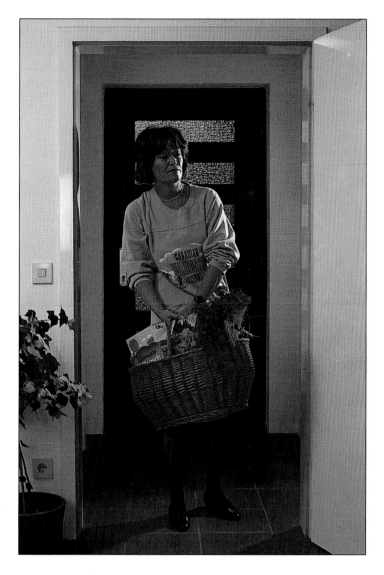

(Above) Everyday activities such as heavy lifting can bring on back pain.

BITES AND STINGS

Insect bites and stings respond well to essential oils. The antiseptic and anti-inflammatory ones help reduce swelling, itchiness and inflammation.

Best Oils: chamomile, lavender, marigold, peppermint, tea tree, basil, citronella (soothing, anti-inflammatory, antiseptic).

BLISTERS

(*see* BURNS)

BREATHING PROBLEMS

Breathing problems caused by bronchitis, influenza and sinusitis are often characterised by the excessive production of mucus, continual coughing, a tight chest and laboured breathing. Essential oils can relax the chest, soothe coughing and breathing and help reduce the congestion.

WARNING: If you suffer from asthma or have a history of serious breathing problems do not use essential oils unless you first consult your doctor.

Best oils: angelica, myrrh (coughs); cedarwood, marjoram, sandalwood (soothing, calming); eucalyptus, peppermint (decongestant); pine, tea tree, rosemary (anti-viral).

BRUISES

A bruise shows that tissue has been injured, usually by a bump or knock. The purple, black or yellow discoloration, which remains long after the initial pain has gone, is due to blood seepage from damaged capillaries.

Best Oils: camphor and clary sage (warming, increases circulation); geranium, calendula, marjoram (soothing); lavender, cypress (anti-inflammatory).

BUNIONS

A bunion is a painful inflammation of the joint between the big toe and the foot, due to long-term aggravation – usually from badly fitting shoes.

Best Oils: peppermint (refreshing, soothing); cypress (anti-inflammatory); lemon (circulation boosting).

BURNS

Burns are caused when skin touches something hot. The resulting blisters and inflammation are very susceptible to infection. The anti-bacterial, anti-viral and antiseptic properties of essential oils help protect the area while new skin grows and help speed up the natural healing process.

Best Oils: lavender, tea tree (soothing, healing, antiseptic, both can be applied undiluted to burnt skin immediately); chamomile, geranium, marigold, rose (soothing, healing).

CELLULITE

Cellulite, the bane of many women's lives, is a lumpy, dimpled, orange-peel textured to skin on thighs, bottom and backs of arms. It is thought to be caused by a build-up of fluid and toxins in the tissues, due to poor circulation and hormonal fluctuations. Regular massage with essential oils can help to smooth the lumpy appearance of the skin.

Best Oils: juniper, geranium (detoxifying); rosemary, fennel (diuretic); bay, cypress, lemon, lime, spruce, cedarwood (circulation boosting); lavender, sage, patchouli (decongestant).

CHICKEN POX

The dreaded disease of childhood, with itchy spots that must not be scratched. Essential oils help tremendously by reducing the itchiness and stopping infection of the pox themselves.

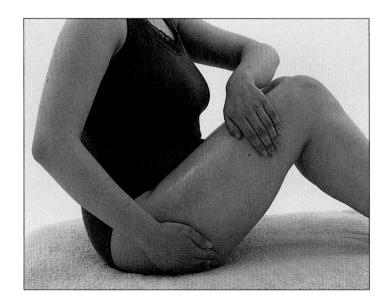

(Above) Detoxifying oils can help to break down the lumpy appearance of cellulite.

Best oils: tea tree, eucalyptus, bergamot, lavender (soothing, antiseptic, healing); chamomile (soothing, anti-itch).

CHILBLAINS

Chilblains appear as swollen, discoloured veins on the fingers, toes and the backs of legs after exposure to very cold weather.

Best Oils: ginger, spruce, eucalyptus (warming, soothing); cypress, marjoram, rosemary, juniper, tea tree, lemongrass, lemon (circulation boosting).

CIRCULATION, POOR

Poor blood circulation is most commonly due to lack of exercise, standing for long periods, or a sedentary lifestyle. Essential oils can help to boost the blood flow, reduce cellulite, warm over-cold hands or feet and give a fresher, healthy glow to the complexion.

Best Oils: basil, cedarwood, cypress, spruce, ginger, juniper, lemon, lemongrass, lavender, myrrh, pine, peppermint, rosemary, clary sage, bay, ambrette seed, ylang-ylang (stimulate circulation); lime, marigold (varicose veins).

COLDS

The common cold is so infectious it is almost inescapable during winter. Caused by a wide range of ever-changing viruses, symptoms include a high temperature, aches, sore eyes, sore throat, coughing, sneezing and chest and nose congestion. Essential oils can help soothe some of these symptoms, but nothing known to science will cure the cold yet.

Best Oils: peppermint, eucalyptus, lavender, lime, pine, tea tree, lemon, marjoram (decongestant, anti-viral); angelica, thyme, camphor, bay, myrrh, spruce (relieve sinus congestion), laurel (strengthens resistance).

COLD SORES

(*see* HERPES)

COUGHS

An irritating cough caused by anything from dust, cigarette smoke and allergy to the common cold can drive anyone to distraction. Inhaled essential oils are very effective at soothing a cough. In fact, many prepared medications such as Karvol or Vicks Vaporub have aromatherapy oils as their main ingredient.

Best Oils: angelica, atlas cedarwood, eucalyptus, peppermint, myrrh, thyme, sandalwood, spruce (expectorant, anti-viral); frankincense (calming and relaxing); ginger, rosemary (decongestant); pine, cedar, cypress, lemon (anti-viral).

CRAMPS

Cramps, excruciating, involuntary muscle spasm caused by the onset of menstruation, poor circulation, too much exercise or a vitamin deficiency, usually hit hardest at dead of night. Essential oils help warm and relax the tense muscles, ease the pain and, if need be, put you back to sleep.

Best Oils: eucalyptus, lemon, marjoram, mandarin (warming, relaxing); juniper (boosts circulation); jasmine, laurel, tarragon, fennel (for period cramps); ambrette seed, rose, lavender, ylang-ylang, neroli, chamomile (relaxing, soporific).

CUTS AND ABRASIONS

Essential oils are excellent at soothing, disinfecting and healing any minor cuts and skin abrasions from nappy rash to shaving nicks.

Best Oils: chamomile, bergamot, lavender, citronella, tea tree (anti-bacterial, antiseptic, anti-viral); geranium, marigold (soothing, healing).

DANDRUFF

Dandruff occurs when there is an imbalance of oils at the skin's surface, and is caused by overactive sebaceous glands. It comes in two forms: fine, dry flakes on the scalp, or sticky, oily scales. Both types are itchy, irritating and can often become infected. Essential oils are excellent at treating dandruff and can usually remove all symptoms.

Best Oils: tea tree (anti-inflammatory, oil regulating, antiseptic); bay, birch, juniper, cedarwood, lemon and rosemary (antiseptic, astringent); lavender, geranium, sandalwood (soothing, antiseptic).

DEPRESSION

Life has so many ups and downs that most of us find our happy moments are balanced by moments of depression. Feeling gloomy is quite normal, but it can make you sleepless, lethargic and downright miserable. Essential oils are particularly good at altering your mood, since smell is registered in the same part of the brain as memories, moods and emotions.

Best Oils: clary sage, sandalwood, geranium, lavender, ylang-ylang (relaxing, uplifting); jasmine, rosewood, neroli, rose, mimosa, bergamot (energising, uplifting); frankincense (for confidence); myrrh (dispels dark moods).

DERMATITIS, ECZEMA, PSORIASIS

Allergenic skin inflammations are becoming more common every year. Perhaps this increase is due to modern living, since stress, anxiety, fatigue and pollution worsen the problem. Essential oils are excellent skin-soothers and healers and can help calm many of the symptoms, particularly inflammation, itchiness and infection.

Best Oils: birch, bergamot, cedarwood, chamomile, cypress, violet (soothing, anti-inflammatory); lavender, geranium, myrrh (healing); marigold (contact dermatitis, psoriasis); sandalwood (extra-dry skin).

FATIGUE

More people complain more of being tired than just about anything else. Too much work, too many demands and stresses, and too little leisure or relaxation are probably to blame. Essential oils are very helpful as they can relax both mind and body in a way that makes you ready for fun rather than sleep.

Best Oils: ambrette seed, eucalyptus, lemongrass, rosemary, peppermint, thyme, ginger, lemon (stimulating); basil, bergamot, clary sage, galbanum, jasmine, lavender (de-stressing, uplifting); fennel, orange, patchouli, geranium, frankincense (gently relaxing).

FLUID RETENTION

Men only seem to suffer from fluid retention after a long aeroplane journey. Most women suffer from it either during menstruation or pregnancy, or simply from being on their feet all day. The swelling can be reduced by massaging with the right essential oils.

WARNING: many essential oils should not be used during pregnancy (see page 69). Consult your doctor first.

Best Oils: birch, juniper, rosemary, fennel (diuretic); cypress (relieves pre-menstrual swelling); mandarin, patchouli, geranium, spruce (stimulating, boost circulation).

FUNGAL INFECTIONS

(*see* ATHLETE'S FOOT *and* THRUSH)

HAIR LOSS

Temporary hair loss often happens after extreme stress, sudden shock, a few months after childbirth or illness. or because of taking some medications. Permanent hair loss, or baldness, is usually inherited. Essential oils can help with thinning hair but, unfortunately, can do nothing to restore a bare scalp.

Best Oils: rosemary, bay, ylang-ylang (rejuvenating, circulation stimulators); lavender, cedarwood (tonic and stimulant); sage, yarrow (promotes hair growth).

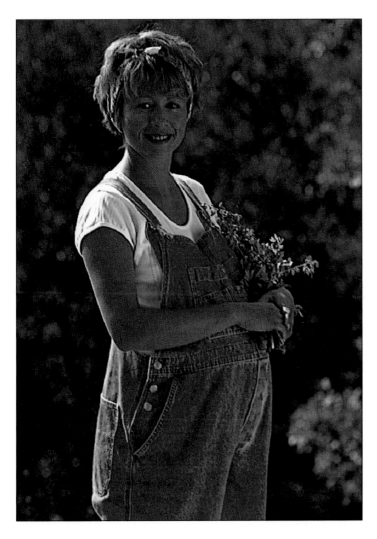

(Above) During pregnancy, fluid retention can be treated with essential oils such as birch or patchouli.

Best Oils: tea-tree, lemon, lavender, geranium (astringent, oil regulators); rosemary, bay, cypress (cleansing, tonic).

HAIR, dry, split

Dry hair can be smoothed down and moisturised with a weekly aromatherapy scalp massage (see page 115). The best carrier oil is avocado or olive oil. Warm 30ml (1fl oz/6 tsps) of carrier oil first, add five drops of the chosen essential oil, then apply. Leave overnight before shampooing out.

Best Oils: chamomile (for blonde hair); rosemary, lavender (red, brown hair); bay (dark hair); tea tree, bergamot (dandruff).

HANGOVER

The morning after too much alcohol, soothe the headache, nausea and lethargy with an aromatherapy bath. Lie back with a neck pillow made from an ice pack and drink lots of glasses of water.

Best Oils: geranium, rose, lavender, neroli (soothing, uplifting); peppermint, lemon (clears the head, energises, reduces nausea).

HAIR, Greasy

Greasy hair lies flat to the head, looks lank and is caused by over-active sebaceous glands in the hair follicles. Hormonal changes brought about by puberty, menstruation, pregnancy and menopause, and stress definitely make the problem worse. An essential oil scalp massage (see page 115) can help by regulating oil production without being too astringent or drying the scalp.

HEADACHE

Headaches may be a sign that the head has had enough. Too much thinking, tension, noise, lights and action don't help, but essential oils do, if you lie in a darkened room and inhale them (see page 95). Or if you can bear it, have a gentle scalp massage (see page 115).

Best Oils: eucalyptus, peppermint, lemongrass (clear the head); lavender, violet, ambrette, rose, chamomile (relaxing, analgesic), frankincense, clary sage, thyme (relieve tension).

HERPES

The herpes virus causes cold sores of the mouth, shingles and genital herpes, and there is no known cure for the painful, recurrent blisters. However, some essential oils can help soothe them and speed up healing.

Best Oils: tea tree, marigold, bergamot, lavender, lemon (healing, anti-viral); chamomile (soothing); eucalyptus and patchouli (antiseptic).

HOUSEHOLD CLEANSERS

Many of today's household cleansers and chemical disinfectants contain essential oils, chosen not only for their fresh, clean smell, but also their antiseptic, anti-fungal and anti-bacterial properties. Think of a pine disinfectant or lemon washing-up liquid. Pine and lemon are two of the most common germ-killing aromatherapy oils. For ways to use the best disinfectant essential oils around the home, see page 99.

Best Oils: lavender, geranium, tea-tree, chamomile, bergamot, citronella, lemon, lime, lemongrass, thyme, eucalyptus, peppermint, pine.

INDIGESTION

Indigestion, heartburn and flatulence are usually the results of eating too quickly and too much, eating a spicy, rich diet, or going for long periods without any food at all. Essential oils massaged into the stomach using slow, circular, clockwise strokes can bring relief. Or try inhaling the aromas from a tissue.

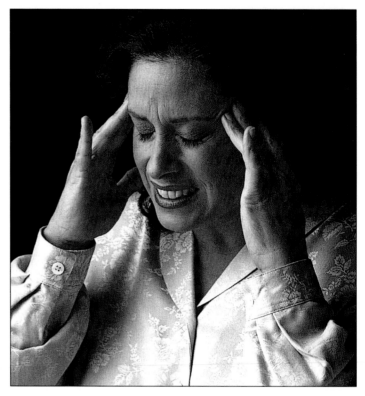

(Above) Headaches are sometimes your body's way of protesting at too much stress or noise.

Best Oils: angelica, fennel, lavender, peppermint, marjoram, tarragon (aches, digestives); ambrette, mandarin (warming, relaxing).

INFLUENZA

Influenza is a more serious viral infection than the common cold and puts most people to bed for a couple of days. Essential oils can soothe some of the symptoms and prevent the virus taking too firm a hold on the 'flu-ravaged body.

Best Oils: eucalyptus, lime, rosemary, peppermint, (clear head congestion); pine, tea-tree (anti-viral); thyme, spruce, marjoram, (expectorant, decongestant); laurel, orange (boost the immune system).

INSECT REPELLENTS

(see BITES AND STINGS)

Insects can take over the entire house in summer, marching out of cracks and crevices, hopping across carpets, flying through windows and all hoping to land on a nice warm bit of skin or clothing. Essential oils make excellent natural, fragrant, non-toxic insecticides that terrify anything small with more than two legs. For how to use them in the home, see page 103.

Best Oils: camphor, lemongrass (moths and most other insects); citronella (mosquitoes); basil, tea-tree, thyme (ants, fleas and most flying insects).

INSOMNIA

(see also STRESS)

Not being able to sleep is deeply irritating, exhausting and distressing, but lying there counting sheep and worrying about it won't help. Use the time to enjoy an aromatherapy bath. You will find that oils with calming, sedative qualities are the most effective.

Best Oils: basil, chamomile, cypress, geranium, lavender, mandarin, neroli, rose, mimosa, petitgrain, marjoram, valerian, jasmine, sandalwood, ylang-ylang, yarrow (calming, sedative).

JETLAG

It seems funny to think that aeroplane travel used to be considered glamorous. Now when most people think of air travel, they think of jet lag, that disorienting experience when you can't sleep at your destination, can't walk off the plane, have swollen feet, dehydrated skin, loss of appetite, can't finish sentences, can't find your baggage ... and all this at the start of your holiday! Essential oils to the rescue. To help adjust to time

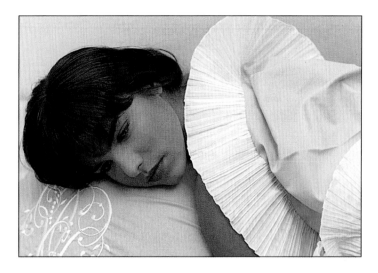

(Above) Sprinkle a few drops of your favourite soothing oil on your sheets for a restful night's sleep.

differences faster, use lavender oil when you land and want to stay awake, and geranium when you want to go to sleep.

Best Oils: lavender (reviving); geranium (relaxing, calming); cypress (for swelling); peppermint (head clearing).

MEASLES

The irritating, itchy rash and bad temper that go with measles can transform even the most angelic child into a miserable little moaner. And when adults get measles, the symptoms are magnified a hundred times. To soothe the skin, gently massage in the right essential oil.
Best Oils: bergamot, lavender, eucalyptus, tea-tree (soothing, antiseptic, uplifting); chamomile (anti-itch, relaxing).

MENOPAUSE

The menopause starts with the natural reduction of oestrogen and progesteron hormones, signalling the end of the childbearing years. It begins at any time from 40 to 60 years, and while many women notice little change, others suffer from a huge selection of unpleasant symptoms, from hot flushes and lack of confidence to abdominal pain and deep depression.

Best Oils: chamomile, rose (rebalancing); lavender, cypress, geranium (regulate hormone production); peppermint, clary sage, ylang-ylang anti-depressant).

MIGRAINE

(*see* HEADACHES)

NAPPY RASH

(*see* CUTS AND ABRASIONS)

NAUSEA

The only thing worse than feeling sick is actually being sick. Common triggers include a rich or spicy meal, contaminated food, a rotten smell, stress, fear, the motion of travel, pregnancy or migraine. A little essential oil inhaled from a tissue helps tremendously.

WARNING: If you are pregnant and are suffering from nausea, see the list of essential oils to be avoided on page 69, and consult your doctor before using aromatherapy to treat the condition.

Best Oils: peppermint, lemon, ginger, mandarin (settle the stomach).

PERSPIRATION

Excessive perspiration or sweatiness can be controlled by using essential oils which are regulating, deodorising, cooling and anti-bacterial. For ways of

using the oils, see page 83.

Best Oils: bergamot, citronella (reduce excessive perspiration); lemongrass, lavender, thyme (anti-bacterial and deodorising).

PMT

(*see also* CRAMPS)

Pre-menstrual tension is the name for a group of symptoms triggered by hormonal changes any time from two days to two weeks before a period. Some women suffer badly with fluid retention in the breasts and abdomen, headaches, nausea, spotty skin, irrational behaviour, moodiness and depression. Essential oils used for bath or massage can help lift the spirits and soothe many of the physical symptoms.

Best Oils: geranium, lavender, rose, chamomile, sandalwood (calming, balancing hormones); bergamot, jasmine, juniper, clary sage (emotionally uplifting); cypress, fennel, tarragon, laurel (fluid retention, cramps); peppermint (energising).

RESPIRATORY INFECTIONS

(*see* BREATHING PROBLEMS and COUGHS)

RHEUMATISM

Rheumatism causes pain in the muscles, ligaments and soft connective tissue around the joints, usually knees, ankles, hips and wrists. Essential oils help soothe the inflammation, relax the tissue and warm the muscles.

Best Oils: angelica, birch, rosemary, juniper, cypress, lavender, eucalyptus, lemon (anti-inflammatory); chamomile (analgesic); angelica, thyme, ginger, lime, pine spruce, marjoram (warming, relaxing).

SEXUAL PROBLEMS

When you jump into bed to sleep rather than to play, you know your life has reached a point where tension and tiredness have taken over from passion. Essential oils are very good at removing the stress and letting you choose whether you want to be sensual or sleepy.

Best Oils: ylang-ylang, clary sage, ginger, jasmine, neroli, patchouli (relaxing, sensual aphrodisiacs); rose, rosewood (romantic, aphrodisiac); sandalwood, geranium (relaxing, uplifting).

SKIN

Essential oils are perfect for day-to-day skincare, because they are rapidly absorbed, penetrate deeply, are easy, aromatic and pleasant to use, are very effective at treating all skin problems and are inexpensive.

Mature Skin

Young skin takes about 30 days to renew itself, but as we get older, this natural process slows and skin loses its soft youthful bloom. Stress, smoking, pollution, alcohol, too much sun and not enough exercise, all help cause premature wrinkling and skin ageing. Essential oils can keep skin smooth and supple longer, and make excellent moisturisers.

Best Oils: rose, neroli, orange, geranium, lavender, frankincense, ylang-ylang, rosemary (skin rejuvenators); chamomile, galbanum (soothing, healing).

Thread Veins

Thread veins are tiny red lines which appear on the skin of cheeks and legs. They're caused by poor circulation, sun or wind exposure and excessive alcohol.

Best Oils: rose, chamomile, geranium (anti-inflammatory, soothing); marigold, cypress, violet,

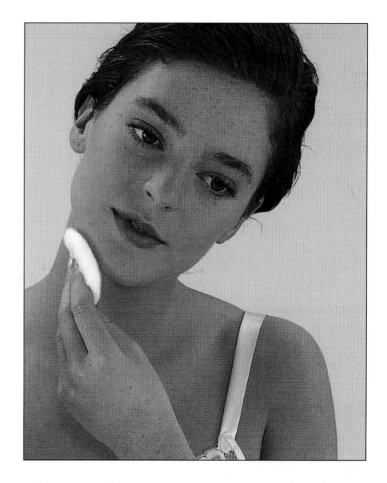

(Above) Aromatherapy moisturisers are easy to make and to use.

lemon, lime, orange, yarrow (vascular constrictors, calming).

Dry/Sensitive Skin

Dry skin can be due to under-active sebaceous glands, too much sun or wind, central heating, alcohol or a bad skincare routine. Soothing, moisturising essential oils can protect and hydrate skin simultaneously.

Best Oils: rose, sandalwood, neroli, marigold, geranium (moisturising); jasmine, lavender, chamomile, violet (sensitive skin); myrrh, tea-tree, patchouli (cracked, rough skin).

Greasy/blemished Skin

With greasy skin, the sebaceous glands are over-

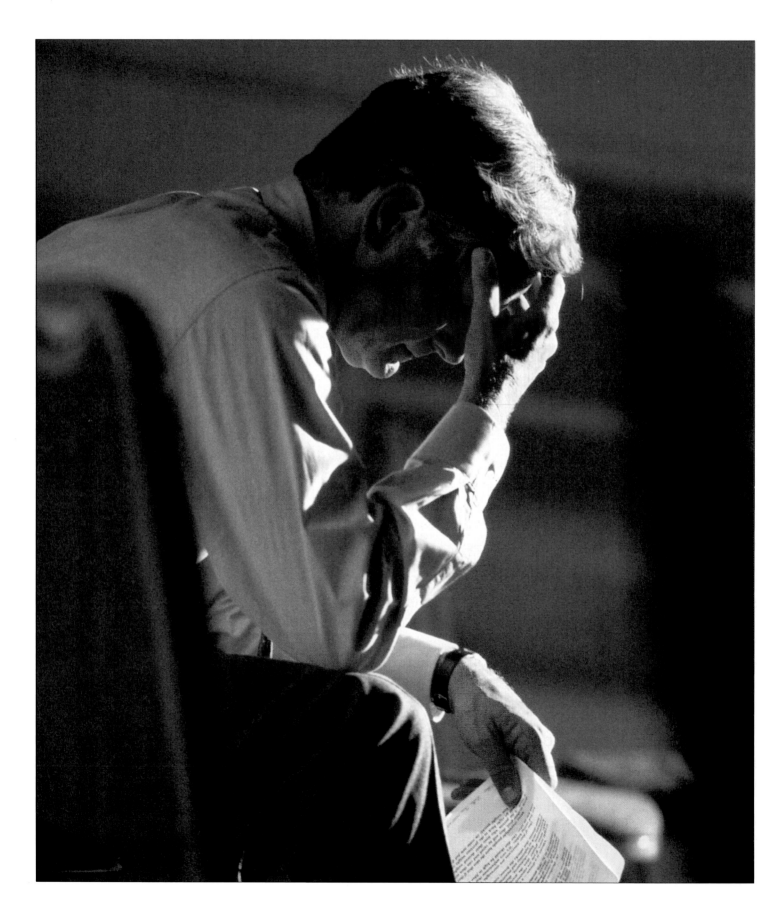

productive and excess oil causes spots, blackheads and open pores. The mildly astringent and healing essential oils are very effective and sometimes regulate skin's natural oil production.

Best Oils: chamomile (soothing, cleansing); lemon, lime, bergamot, mandarin, cedarwood, juniper, geranium (rebalancing, antiseptic); neroli, lavender (healing); lemongrass, petitgrain (open pores); violet, patchouli, thyme (blackheads).

STRESS

Stress is a part of our complicated, modern lifestyle and is caused by excessive demands on our time and energies. It shows as muscular aches and pains, allergies, insomnia, anxiety, depression, nervousness and irritability, and can lead to serious illness. Calming, relaxing and uplifting essential oils help tremendously.

Best Oils: jasmine, basil, neroli, rosewood, geranium, bergamot, sandalwood, ylang-ylang, rose, frankincense, galbanum (anti-stress, uplifting); marjoram, mandarin, clary sage, valerian, lavender, chamomile, patchouli (calming, sedative).

SUNBURN

Sunburn is something we are not meant to get these days, now that we all know that sunbathing ages skin and causes cancers. But if you do burn, essential oils can boost the skin's natural healing process, and soothe and cool the initial burning.

Best Oils: lavender, chamomile, geranium, rose (soothing, anti-inflammatory).

(Left) The symptoms of stress range from muscular pain to allergies and depression.

SWEATINESS

(see PERSPIRATION)

THRUSH, CANDIDA, FUNGAL PROBLEMS

The most useful essential oil for vaginal or genital fungal infections is tea-tree; it has amazing anti-viral, anti-fungal and disinfectant properties that have only recently been discovered. It is safe and non-irritating to sensitive genital tissue. Apply one part essential oil to ten parts warm water and use to bathe the affected area or as a douche. Some other antiseptic oils can help to soothe, heal and reduce itchiness.

Best Oils: tea-tree (anti-fungal); juniper, lavender, myrrh, sandalwood (antiseptic).

THREAD VEINS

(see SKIN)

TRAVEL SICKNESS

Travel sickness is usually caused by the motion of travelling by air, sea or land, but the nausea can also be due to an actual fear of travelling.

Best Oils: peppermint, ginger, lemon, mandarin (calming, settle the stomach); bergamot (uplifting, soothing).

VARICOSE VEINS

(see CIRCULATION, POOR

WRINKLES

(see SKIN, Mature)

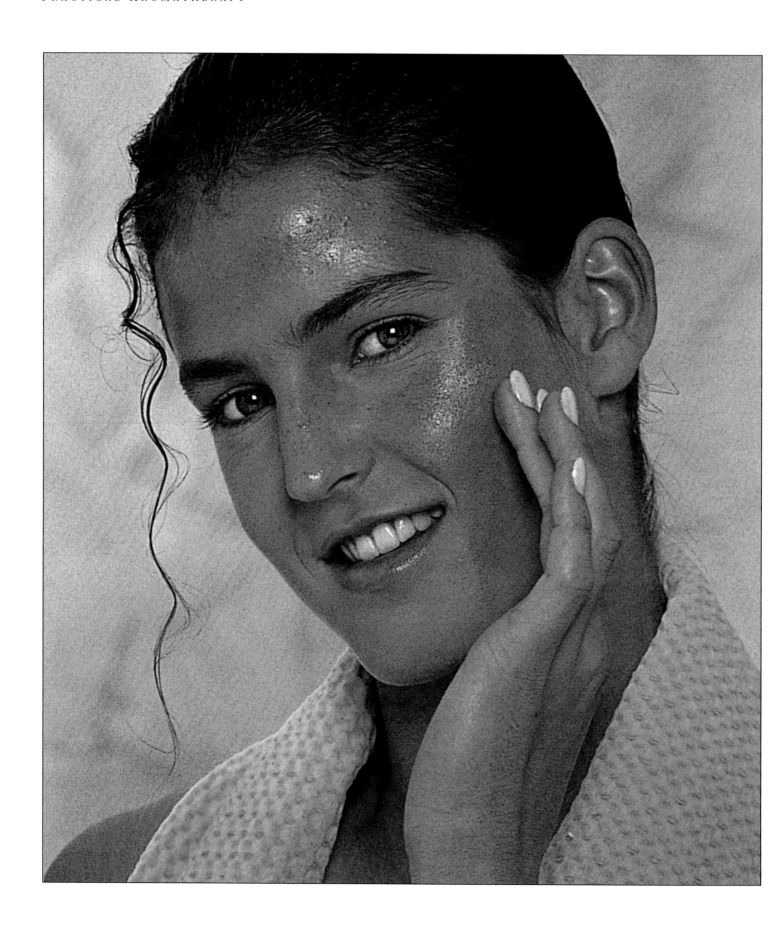

How to Use Essential Oils

Essential oils are potent and should never be used unless they have been diluted first, either in water, for the bath, or with a plain carrier oil, for massage. Applying double the dose of essential oils does not mean you get twice the benefits: some oils in excess will make you feel nauseous, others are highly toxic. And all of them are so powerful that they are measured in drops.

To use essential oils properly, safely and for maximum benefit, always follow instructions for individual recipes exactly. Make sure you read the list of warnings on page 69. And since essential oils are quite expensive (a gram of jasmine, for instance, costs almost as much as a gram of gold), make sure that you dilute, blend and store oils in the following way so that they last as long as possible without deteriorating in quality.

DILUTING ESSENTIAL OILS

Essential oils are always measured in drops. They are usually sold in tiny, 10-ml (½ fluid-oz) dark glass bottles and most have droppers built into the caps. But if they don't, you can use an eye-dropper or pipette to measure out droplets. If you are using more than one oil, wash the dropper thoroughly in between or you will mix the oils and ruin their individual aromas.

Essential oils are so volatile they evaporate rapidly so measure drops out quickly and accurately. If you accidently spill the bottle, blot the oil up immediately with paper towels, tissue or toilet roll, then wash it with warm water and detergent. If you just leave the oil it will evaporate through the room and may make you feel sick or headachy if it is too potent. All recipes in this book specify exact drops of essential oils. But if you are mixing your own combinations, the general rules for safe dilution are as follows:

For Massage
15 – 20 drops essential oil in 60ml (2 fl oz/12 tsp) carrier oil
7 – 10 drops essential oil in 30ml (1 fl oz/6 tsp) carrier oil
3 – 5 drops essential oil in 15ml (½ fl oz/3 tsp) carrier oil

For Bath
8 – 10 drops maximum essential oils in any one bath

(Left) Our favourite fragrances evoke positive memories and feelings.

BLENDING ESSENTIAL OILS

For massage or application anywhere on the skin, essential oils should first be mixed with a carrier (or base) oil. Any of the pure, cold-pressed plant oils will do, as these not only dilute essential oils so they are safe, but also help spread them evenly, slow down their evaporation rate, and increase their absorption into skin.

When blending essential oils, first measure out the carrier oil and put it in a ceramic bowl for immediate use, or a glass bottle if you are going to store it. Then add the drops of essential oil and mix them well. If you are making enough to keep for repeated use, make sure you label your bottle clearly with the number of essential oil drops in the mix.

It is important to choose a pure, good quality vegetable oil as carrier for your essential oils. Mineral oil (usually called baby oil) is not a good carrier because it has a low penetrating ability.

Best Carrier Oils for Body
grapeseed

sweet almond

sunflower

safflower

peanut

soya

sesame *(for stretch marks)*

•

Best Carrier Oils for Face
sweet almond

peach kernel

apricot kernel

jojoba

avocado

evening primrose *(for wrinkles)*

STORING ESSENTIAL OILS

Pure essential oils should be stored in a cool place, in dark glass, airtight bottles, out of direct sunshine, and out of reach of children. This way, they should keep in perfect condition for up to a year.

Once essential oils are diluted with a carrier oil, they will keep for up to six months if you add the contents of a vitamin E capsule, or one teaspoon of wheatgerm oil. This acts as an anti-oxidant and will help preserve your mixture. Otherwise, keep it in the fridge so the carrier oil doesn't go rancid. It is always best to blend oils for aromatherapy in small amounts so that they are as fresh and potent as possible.

COMBINING ESSENTIAL OILS

When it comes to creating your own essential oil recipes, for pleasure or treatment, the main rule is to keep them simple until you have had some practise.

You will find that some essential oils cancel each other out, while some clash. Others help one another therapeutically: for example, chamomile's anti-inflammatory action is strengthened by lavender. And some, especially lavender and rose, go with anything.

The Ten Best Mixers
bergamot

lavender

chamomile

neroli

frankincense

rose

geranium

sandalwood

jasmine

ylang-ylang

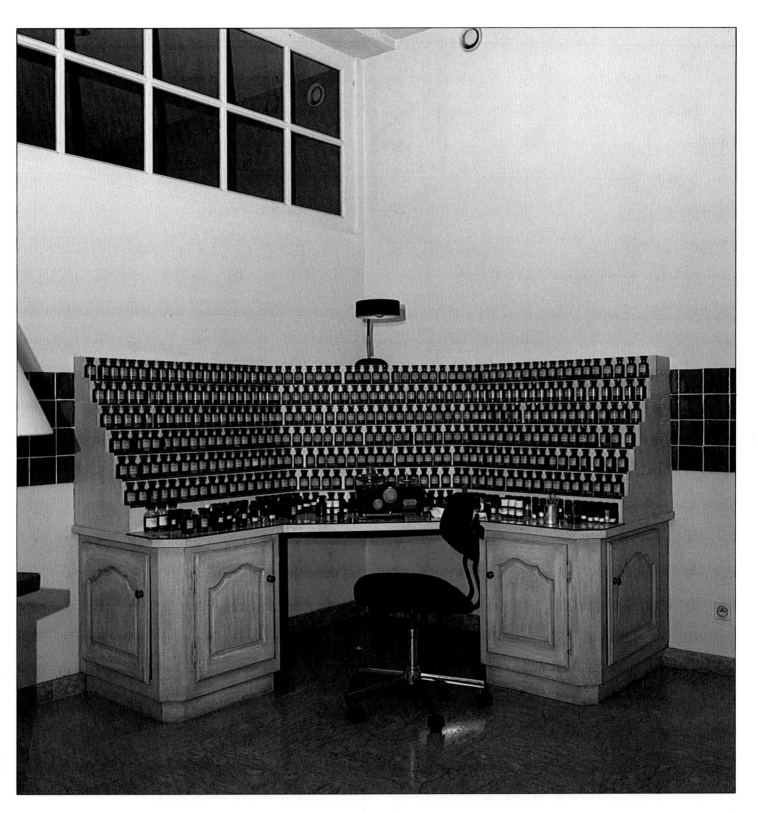

*(Above) In this perfumery in Grasse, the essential oils
are carefully stored in airtight bottles.*

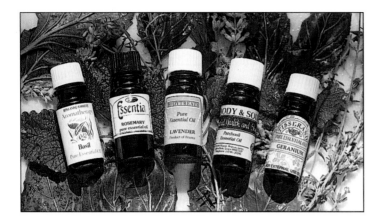

(Above) Blends of only two or three oils are often best.

Male Favourites	Female Favourites
basil	bergamot
bergamot	geranium
eucalyptus	jasmine
frankincense	lavender
jasmine	neroli
lavender	patchouli
lemon	peppermint
patchouli	rose
pine	sage
sandalwood	ylang-ylang

LEARNING TO MIX

When you first start mixing your own combinations, use the chart on page 46 for an instant reference on which oils work well together. Also remember that less is best. Use only three oils per blend for most combinations. Occasionally you can use four, but only if they are from the same fragrance category (see page 14): for instance, four floral essential oils, such as lavender, neroli, ylang-ylang and rose.

Always try your combination before you mix it so you don't waste essential oils. The best way is to cut up some long strips of blotting paper. Apply one drop of each oil to the tip of one blotter strip if you are going to be using oils in equal amounts. If one oil will dominate your recipe more than the others, put two drops of the dominant oil on the tip of the blotter. Then hold the strips together by the bottom end and fan the oily tips backwards and forwards under your nose while you inhale.

Let your nose be the judge, and if you like the combination, go ahead and mix it. Since our favourite fragrances are determined by the memories and feelings they evoke as much as by their actual odour, aromatherapy is a very personal thing. If you are making a combination for someone else, ensure you test it on them first with blotting paper, because although you may adore it, they might not.

WARNINGS FOR HOME USE

Stimulating your sense of smell, your moods, behaviour and mental and physical wellbeing are just some of the miracles essential oils are capable of. Using them is also a great pleasure, as long as you use them properly. Here are the basic rules to ensure you that you will have no problems.

■ Essential oils are potent: only ever measure them out in drops.

■ Never apply undiluted essential oils to skin, apart from lavender for minor cuts and burns, and tea tree for spots, fungal infections, etc, and even these two should be used in moderation.

■ Don't take essential oils internally. A professional aromatherapist may prescribe oral treatment: otherwise it is unsafe.

■ Increasing the dose of essential oils does not increase their effectiveness. In fact, some oils in large amounts are toxic.

For therapeutic use to treat common ailments, only apply essential oils as instructed and always seek medical advice if symptoms persist.

Keep essential oils out of reach of children: if any splashes in an eye, rinse it out with a few drops of pure, sweet, almond oil rather than using water, and seek medical advice.

Don't shower or bath for two hours after an aromatherapy massage. It takes that long for some oils to fully penetrate skin.

It is best not to use glass bottles for an aromatherapy massage mix for once you have oily hands, glass bottles are very slippery to hold. Use a. bowl instead and dip your hands into it.

Don't store essential oils, pure or diluted, in plastic containers or they will become contaminated.

Don't expose skin to sunshine for six hours if you have used a citrus oil. After exposure to the sun they become photo-toxic and can cause skin irritation.

ESSENTIAL EQUIPMENT

10-ml (½-fluid-oz) dark glass bottles with stoppered caps for storing pure essential oils

four eye-droppers/pipettes (or one if you wash it thoroughly after each use)

a small funnel for pouring carrier oils into bottles

large, dark glass, stoppered bottles for storing combinations of oils or a ceramic bowl for immediate use. Never use metal containers or bowls.

strips of blotting paper

Oils to be Used in Moderation

basil
bay
camphor
fennel
ginger
laurel
sage tarragon
thyme
valerian

•

Oils that are Photo-toxic

angelica
bergamot
citronella
ginger
lemon
lime
mandarin

•

Oils to be Avoided in Pregnancy

angelica
citronella
laurel
rosemary
thyme
basil
fennel
marjoram
sage
yarrow
cedarwood
juniper
myrrh
tarragon

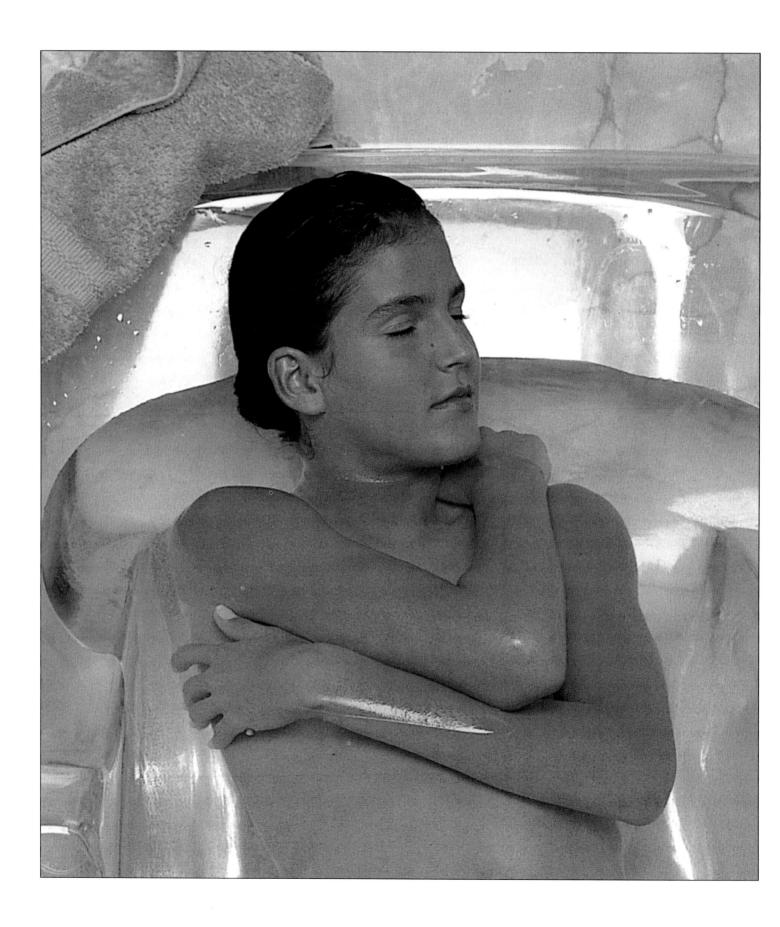

ESSENTIAL OILS IN THE BATH

Cleopatra bathed in asses' milk, the ancients Romans socialised in
hot pools for hours, and Mary, Queen of Scots preferred to soak in a tub of hot wine.
Today, some of us bathe in salt water, others in ice-cold water and others use jets,
steam, sprays, spurts or gurgles. No matter what, the splashing water
and steam combined with a relaxing, warm soak make bathtime
the most restful part of the day in a mad world.

But when you add essential oils to your bath, you transform a pleasurable experience
into a heavenly one. It is the most relaxing aromatherapy treatment possible.
Because you're in a warm, steamy room, the oils release more aroma molecules than
during massage, and as you lie soaking in the hot water it softens skin
and speeds up oil absorption, allowing the essential oils to work
their magic more potently on both mind and body.

Also, since the aroma is so much stronger in warm, steamy air, if you use more
than one essential oil you'll notice that it is like sniffing a bunch of flowers.
If you keep your eyes closed, not only can you smell the whole bouquet, but you
can name all the blooms individually. The effect is caused by heat making the
individual oils come in waves, so you can smell them singly and
combined, with the result that they smell so different
and divine, you'll hardly recognise them.

(Left) Bath oils can revive or relax, soothe skin or relieve aches.

THE AROMA BATH

To get the best from an aromatic bath, make sure that everything is as comfortable and cosy as possible before you get undressed. And remember that you can use essential oils in the bath to give almost any effect. They are particularly good to energise or relax, to soothe itchy, dry or sunburnt skin, relieve muscular aches, PMT or cramps, or treat a cold, hangover or headache. In summer, floral or citrus baths are very refreshing. In winter, green, spicy or woody ones are the most warming and relaxing.

Ten Best Bath Oils

If you want to add a single oil to your bath the best all-rounders at any time of the year are:

5 drops bergamot *(for melancholy, depression)*
7 drops chamomile *(for insomnia, itchy skin)*
8 drops frankincense *(sedative, calming, mood sweetening)*
10 drops geranium *(relaxing, but uplifting, energising)*
8 drops jasmine *(for apathy, stress, fatigue)*
10 drops lavender *(relaxing, soothing, positive)*
8 drops neroli *(hypnotic, anti-depressant)*
5 drops patchouli *(energising, invigorating)*
10 drops rose *(romantic, happiness, pleasure)*
8 drops sandalwood *(intimate, sensual, mellowing)*

Vital Comforters
- a warm room
- soft lighting
- a neck pillow or rolled towel
- soothing eye pads
- lots of large, warm towels
- the telephone off the hook

Bathtime Basics

When adding essential oils, make sure that the bathroom door is closed and taps are turned off to keep as much scent in the room as possible. Add essential oils gently, drop by drop, so they float on the surface of the water, and then they will coat your skin and mix as you step into the tub.

Although you will only smell the aroma for a few minutes, don't be tempted to add extra oil. The human nose soon gets accustomed to the same smell and stops registering it, but the oils will keep evaporating for 15 minutes or more.

Also smaller amounts of essential oils often have greater effect than larger amounts, so don't be fooled into thinking double the amount will get rid of your headache twice as quickly. It won't, and if you use oils in too strong a concentration, you risk irritating skin.

How Many Drops

In general, add up to ten drops of essential oil for one bath, but some of the stronger-smelling oils such as eucalyptus, peppermint, bay, basil, lime, lemon, thyme and rosemary need only five drops per bath to be effective. Use a single oil alone, or mix up to three different ones per bath, but don't put any more than this for they will only cancel one another's benefits out.

Choosing Oils

When choosing oils, use ones with similar or complementary effects. They fall into three main categories – stimulating, relaxing, or therapeutic (see the chart on page 50). Therapeutic oils may be added to either of the other two types, but mixing relaxing and stimulating oils together may cancel out any good they do on their own.

If you need help deciding which specific oils to use, refer back to the at-a-glance chart for mixing oils (see page 46) and the directory of common problems (see page 52). To inspire you to experiment further on your own, here is a selection of tried and tested bathtime recipes that soothe body, mind and soul in one go.

RELAXING BATHS

IN SUMMER OR HOT WEATHER
4 drops lavender, 4 drops neroli and 2 drops geranium
– OR –
4 drops mandarin, 4 drops geranium and 2 drops pine

IN WINTER OR COLD WEATHER
3 drops sandalwood, 3 drops ylang- ylang and
2 drops pine
– OR –
4 drops patchouli, 2 drops ginger and 2 drops
frankincense

AFTER A HARD DAY
5 drops rose and 5 drops lavender –
– OR –
3 drops chamomile, 3 drops geranium and
2 drops patchouli

FOR HER
3 drops rose, 3 drops jasmine and 4 drops neroli
– OR –
3 drops ylang-ylang, 3 drops sandalwood amd
3 drops jasmine

FOR HIM
3 drops pine, 2 drops chamomile and 2 drops lemon
– OR –
4 drops frankincense, 2 drops basil or
3 drops sandalwood

INVIGORATING BATHS

IN SUMMER OR HOT WEATHER
2 drops each basil, patchouli and juniper
– OR –
3 drops rosemary, 3 drops mint and 3 drops lemon

IN WINTER OR COLD WEATHER
3 drops eucalyptus, 3 drops clary sage and 2 drops mint
– OR –
3 drops petitgrain, 3 drops bergamot and
2 drops lemon

AFTER A HARD DAY
5 drops patchouli and 4 drops mint
– OR –
4 drops rosemary, 4 drops thyme and 2 drops mint

FOR HER
4 drops ylang-ylang and 4 drops petitgrain
– OR –
2 drops each mint, clary sage and basil

FOR HIM
3 drops rosemary, 3 drops mint and 2 drops juniper
– OR –
4 drops each thyme and basil

THERAPEUTIC BATHS

BATH FOR COUGHS AND COLDS
3 drops pine, 2 drops lemon and 2 drops tea tree
– OR –
3 drops eucalyptus, 3 drops lavender and 2 drops mint

BATH FOR DRY OR ITCHY SKIN
5 drops lavender and 5 drops chamomile
– OR –
4 drops rose, 4 drops chamomile and 2 drops jasmine

BATH FOR ACHES AND PAINS
4 drops eucalyptus, 3 drops clary sage and
3 drops thyme
– OR –
3 drops marjoram, 2 drops ginger and
4 drops rosemary

BATH FOR SLEEPLESSNESS
2 drops each ylang-ylang, rose, lavender and neroli
– OR –
3 drops chamomile, 2 drops camphor, 2 drops juniper

BATH FOR HEADACHE / HANGOVER
5 drops each rose and lavender
(plus some ice folded in a towel as a neck pillow)
– OR –
2 drops mint, 2 drops lemon and 4 drops marjoram

ESSENTIAL AQUATHERAPY

As well as getting a therapeutic effect from the essential oils you use, you can change the type of bath just by altering the water: very hot or very cold for an in-and-out quick bath; tepid or warm water for a good, long, skin-wrinkling soak. You can use aquatherapy before aromatherapy. A plain bath without essential oils will soften skin and warm and relax muscles to make an aromatherapy massage or body moisturiser afterwards even more effective.

Cold water stimulates, tepid makes you sleepy, warm is relaxing and hot leaves you weak and floppy. So the best time for a relaxing bath is after dark, at the end of a hard day. An invigorating one is good first thing in the morning, to wake you up. Or if you use aquatherapy cleverly, you can combine the two water temperatures for those occasions when you get home tired, need to relax, but have to have the energy to go out again.

The kindest way to combine hot and cold water, without getting goose bumps, is to start off relaxing in a warm or hot bath. After a good soak, let half the water out, turn on the cold tap and let the bath slowly refill. While the cold water is running, stir the bathwater with your hand and you will feel the hot and cold water separately, in waves swirling round your body. By the time the bath is full, you'll be refreshed and raring to go, but not shivering.

Best Cold Bath Oils

10 drops geranium
5 drops lemon
8 drops mimosa
5 drops peppermint
8 drops violet

•

Best Hot Bath Oils

6 drops chamomile
8 drops frankincense
10 drops lavender
8 drops neroli
6 drops ylang-ylang

Temperature Tips
- A cool bath (65-75°F/18-24°C) is the most invigorating, energising pick-me-up
- A tepid bath (75-85°F/24-30°C) is the most soporific and gentle
- A warm bath (85-95°F/30-35°C) is the most deeply relaxing and soothes aches
- A hot bath (95°F/35°C or more) is slightly debilitating and leaves you weak. Avoid them when you are pregnant or if you have varicose veins, heart problems or high blood pressure

THE AROMATIC SHOWER

Using essential oils under the shower is not quite as therapeutic as using them in the bath. Since the water is always running, a lot of the oil and its aroma goes down the plughole. It is best to use aromatic showers as a way to wake up your mind and body, because it is quite difficult to relax deeply when you're standing up!

> **Best Shower Oils**
> basil
> bergamot
> lemongrass
> lime
> mandarin
> orange
> peppermint
> pine

The best way to avoid wasting essential oils in the shower is to mix them first with a carrier oil, then massage them in before you get under the spray. Or you can dip a sponge into the mixture and rub it over your body while you shower. If you have a deep base to your shower, you can make it more aromatic by blocking up the plug so the oils vaporise in the warm water at the bottom.

THE ESSENTIAL FOOTBATH

The feet suffer more stresses than almost any other part of the body. They have to carry all that weight throughout the day and then maybe dance all night. The best reward you can give them is a soothing foot soak. It warms and relaxes all the tiny support muscles, releases trapped nerves, improves the blood circulation and soothes aches and pains.

The right essential oil will make it even more pleasurable. And since you have to sit while you soak, you get to inhale the aroma molecules and enjoy a moment of stillness in a busy day. All you need is a large basin or square bucket, hot water a warm towel, a comfortable seat at the most relaxing height and the right essential oils. Just add them, drop by drop to the water before you slip your feet in. You need up to eight drops per nine litres (two gallons) of water.

STIMULATING FOOTBATHS

2 drops bay and 4 drops of ginger
– OR –
4 drops citronella and 4 drops angelica

RELAXING FOOTBATHS

5 drops basil
– OR –
3 drops lavender and 3 drops geranium

THERAPEUTIC FOOTBATHS

FOR ACHING FEET
4 drops thyme and 4 drops chamomile
– OR –
4 drops eucalyptus and 3 drops pine

FOR ATHLETE'S FOOT
3 drops birch and 6 drops geranium
– OR –
8 drops tea-tree

EXCESSIVE SWEATING
6 drops lemongrass
– OR –
4 drops bergamot and 4 drops citronella

> **A Mini Bath**
> Footbaths and handbaths are especially helpful if you are elderly or have a disability that prevents you from taking a full aromatherapy bath – or simply if a full bath is impractical for you at any time.

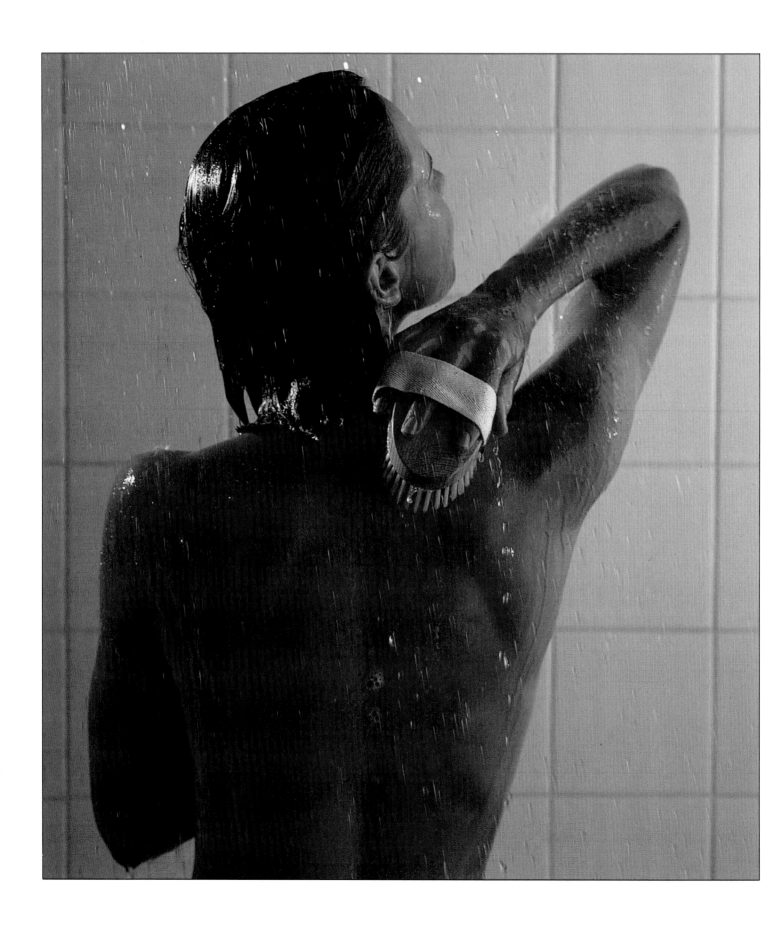

ESSENTIAL OILS FOR THE BODY

Skincare is not something that starts from the neck up. In fact, the skin on
the rest of your body is just the same as that on your face, and as there is more of it,
it needs more attention. Most people would say their bodies weren't
perfect, yet they do very little to improve them.

However, using essential oils on the body achieves more, in less time, than any other
beauty regime. This is because you can treat individual areas with made-to-measure
products that are instantly absorbed, inexpensive and very effective.

Instead of buying an exfoliator to smooth skin, you can make your own and include
an essential oil to break down cellulite at the same time. Or instead of using
an all-over body lotion, you can create one moisturiser with an essential oil to treat
your oily back and another to soothe the dry skin on the rest of your body.

ESSENTIAL MOISTURISERS

An essential-oil moisturiser is undoubtedly the best body treatment available. To apply
essential oils for maximum benefit you need to dilute them with a carrier oil,
not only to stop them being too strong, but also so that they spread evenly,
evaporate slowly and are held on the skin while they're absorbed.
And it is the carrier oil, as much as the aromatic ones you add,
that makes them such good moisturisers.

All moisturising creams work by sealing the surface of your skin to trap the natural
water inside the tissues and stop it evaporating out into the air. As it is the oil,
not water, that gives the moisturising effect, the more oil in
your moisturiser, the better.

This is particularly so with body moisturisers. Legs and arms have few sebaceous
glands (the oil-producing pores that help keep skin naturally soft) and
this is why you so often get rough, dry patches on the feet, knees and elbows.
However the upper back has so many sebaceous glands that
they often block causing spots and greasiness.

(Left) The upper back may need treatment for oiliness.

WHEN TO USE THEM

An essential-oil body treatment is pure oil for maximum moisturisation with the right therapeutic drops added for your needs. And that is all it is. You can use them as much as you like; they're additive-free, simple, pure, non-irritating, very inexpensive and quick and easy to mix.

The best time to apply them is after a bath or shower, when skin is soft, warm, damp and slightly swollen with water. Then, the essential oils are absorbed more rapidly into the skin. If you want to put it to the test, rub a peeled clove of garlic into the sole of your foot after a bath and see how quickly you can smell garlic on your breath.

Since it is ideal to apply body moisturisers morning and night and most of us don't bathe twice a day, the next best way to speed up oil absorption is with massage. When oil is rubbed over skin the friction and body heat warms it, so it almost melts into the body. You can follow a complete routine like the energising top-to-toe self-massage (see page 118) or just rub the oils in using firm, rhythmic palm strokes to create maximum heat and friction.

HOW TO USE THEM

Body moisturisers need to be applied over a very large area of warm skin, so the oils should be well-diluted. Otherwise your body heat can make them so aromatic they are overpowering. Always apply them sparingly so the carrier oil is totally absorbed: if you smear yourself like a sardine, the oil will mark clothes and be wasted.

Mix just enough to last for a few days, for the fresher the ingredients the better the beneficial properties. If you really need to mix a large batch, add the contents of a vitamin E capsule or a teaspoon of wheatgerm oil to act as a natural preservative. The ideal recipe for body moisturisers should have 15 drops of the essential oil in 60ml (2fl oz/12 tsps) carrier oil.

HOW TO BLEND THEM

The right essential-oil body moisturiser depends very much on choosing the right carrier oil. Some are light and instantly absorbed, some are richer and more emollient and some are particularly good for individual skin problems.

Always buy pure, cold-pressed oils as these are the best quality and blend well with essential oils. You should first measure out your chosen carrier oil into a dark glass bottle, then add the essential oils, drop by drop. Always store in a cool, dark place and shake well before use.

Best Carrier Oils

wheat germ
(for scars)

•

sesame
(for stretch marks)

•

apricot kernel, evening primrose
(for wrinkles)

•

safflower, sunflower
(for oily skin)

•

sweet almond
(for normal, itchy or sensitive skins)

•

peanut
(for dry skin)

•

olive oil
(for rough skin)

ESSENTIAL BODY MOISTURISERS

When you're making your own essential-oil body moisturiser, you can decide whether you're adding aroma for pleasure, for treatment – or for both effects. If it is purely for pleasure, let your nose be your guide. It is nice to layer the fragrance, so if you use aromatherapy baths, match your moisturiser to your bath oils. The therapeutic oils can always be applied in tiny amounts just to the particular trouble spots, and then you can use an aromatic mix for the rest of your body. Or if you mix the two, you will feel better and look better in one go.

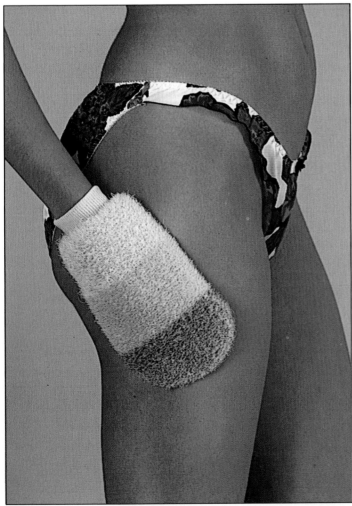

(Above) Use a loofah mitt to massage in oils for cellulite.

Best Aromatic Oils

geranium
jasmine
lavender
mimosa
neroli
rose
sandalwood
violet

•

Best Therapeutic Oils

bergamot
(for oily skin)

•

chamomile
(for itchy skin)

•

cypress
(for cellulite)

•

frankincense
(stretch marks)

•

lavender
(for sensitive skin)

•

myrrh
(for dry skin)

•

rose
(mature skin)

•

tea tree
(cracked, rough skin)

THE BEST COMBINATIONS

To make your own recipes, you need to consult the chart for mixing oils (see page 46) and the chart of essential oil uses (see page 50) to make sure your combinations will smell and work as wonderfully as possible. Since the finished product will cover you from top to toe, remember that the final aroma must be something that delights your nose. If you're unsure, do the blotting paper sniff test (see page 14) to get an idea of the final bouquet before you mix it up. To set you on the right track, here is a selection of excellent body moisturising recipes for you to try.

RICH MOISTURISERS

For Mature Skin
7 drops rose and 4 drops each lavender and sandalwood in 60ml (2fl oz/12 tsps) apricot kernel oil
– OR –
4 drops galbanum, 5 drops geranium and 6 drops lavender in 60ml (2fl oz/12 tsps) sesame oil

For Dry Skin
8 drops myrrh and 7 drops rose in 60ml (2fl oz/12 tsps) peanut oil
– OR –
5 drops each patchouli, sandalwood and jasmine in 60ml (2fl oz/12 tsps) sweet almond oil

For Summer
4 drops each chamomile, lavender and sandalwood in 60ml (2fl oz/12 tsps) peanut oil
– OR –
7 drops each rose and neroli in 60ml (2fl oz/12 tsps) grapeseed oil

For Winter
5 drops each sandalwood, juniper and petitgrain in 60ml (2fl oz/12 tsps) olive oil
– OR –
6 drops lavender, 4 drops frankincense and 4 drops myrrh in 60ml (2fl oz/12 tsps) of sweet almond oil

LIGHT MOISTURISERS

For oily skin
8 drops lavender and 3 drops each lemon and petitgrain in 60 ml (2fl oz/12 tsps)) sunflower oil
– OR –
5 drops each bergamot, chamomile and geranium in 60ml (2fl oz/12 tsps) safflower oil

For Itchy/Sensitive Skin
5 drops rose and 9 drops chamomile in 60ml (2fl oz/12 tsps) sweet almond oil
– OR –
8 drops lavender, 2 drops marigold and 5 drops violet in 60ml (2fl oz/12 tsps) sweet almond oil

For Summer
5 drops each bergamot, geranium, and neroli in 60ml (2fl oz/12 tsps) safflower oil
– OR –
6 drops rose, 4 drops jasmine and 5 drops mimosa in 60ml (2fl oz/12 tsps) sunflower oil

For Winter
4 drops each sandalwood, patchouli and myrrh in 60ml (2fl oz/12 tsps) sweet almond oil
– OR –
6 drops sandalwood and 4 drops each orange and ylang-ylang in 60ml (2fl oz/12 tsps) sunflower oil

OTHER BODY TREATMENTS

The basic carrier-oil/essential-oil body moisturiser mix may be used to create all sorts of other treatment products. If you add some to a little hot water, you get an excellent pre-manicure, nail-softening soak. If you add a grainy ingredient, such as coarse sea salt or roughly chopped almonds, it makes a smoothing and soothing body exfoliator. And if you need to treat a specific area, you can add finely ground oatmeal, kaolin or fuller's earth to thicken the mix and apply it as a body mask.

How to blend them
These products are ideal for treating trouble spots all over the body, and since you can custom blend exactly what you want, and how much, they're also extremely cost-effective.

BODY EXFOLIATOR

For patches of very rough skin
Place 5 heaped tablespoons of coarse sea salt in screw-top glass jar. Add 5ml (0.2fl oz/1tsp) body moisturiser and mix by sprinkling it all over the salt in small droplets. Then shake the jar to mix and leave overnight before use.

Uses: With skin slightly damp, rub it into heels, knees and elbows to remove thick, rough patches of skin. Rinse off with warm water and apply a body moisturiser immediately afterwards.

For dry or coarse skin
Finely blend or chop two tablespoons of fresh almonds and add enough body moisturiser mix to make a smooth paste. Coarsely chop two tablespoons of fresh almonds and mix through the paste. Use immediately.

Uses: With skin slightly damp, rub the paste in circular movements over buttocks, thighs, upper arms, upper back, shoulders or anywhere else that skin is dull. Finish by rubbing in a rich body moisturiser.

BODY PACK

For a small area of skin
Heat 10ml (0.4fl oz/2 tsps) body-moisturiser mix by standing the glass bottle in boiling water. Then mix with finely blended oatmeal to make a thick paste.

Uses: Ideal to spread on a spotty chest or back, or dry patches of skin. Apply the paste while it is still warm for a drawing effect, then rinse off once it has cooled.

For a large area of skin
Combine 60ml (2fl oz/12 tsps) body moisturiser mix with enough dried kaolin or fuller's earth to make a smooth, soft paste. Apply immediately.

Uses: For cellulite, fluid retention or varicose veins, spread the paste thinly over the area and leave it to harden. Rinse off then massage in a body moisturiser.

BODY SOAK

For rough or hard skin
Add 30ml (1fl oz/6 tsps) body-moisturiser mix to a little hot water in a basin. Use immediately.

Uses: Use before a manicure or pedicure. For patches of very hard skin, use a pumice stone immediately after soaking. Finish with a body moisturiser.

For thick, coarse skin
Add 30ml (1fl oz/6 tsps) body-moisturiser mix to a little hot water. Soak a piece of cotton cloth in it until sodden, then wring it out and apply it immediately.

Uses: Ideal for softening elbows, knees or other areas of coarse skin before massaging in a body moisturiser.

TOP-TO-TOE TROUBLE SPOTS

Essential oils are excellent for treating any problems close to the skin as they penetrate it quickly and effectively. All the usual trouble spots from blackheads to stretch marks respond very well, so it is worth persisting by applying the right body oils morning and night for at least two weeks. Here is a selection of recipes for the most common skin and body beauty complaints.

THE FEET

FOR COLD FEET AND POOR CIRCULATION
3 drops each eucalyptus and ginger
in 30ml (1fl oz/6 tsps) olive oil

FOR CALLOUSES AND ROUGH SKIN
3 drops each lavender and sandalwood
in 30ml (1fl oz/6 tsps) olive oil

FOR ATHLETE'S FOOT, WARTS, CORNS
3 drops lemon and 4 drops tea-tree
in 30ml (1fl oz/6 tsps) olive oil

THE KNEES

FOR THICK, COARSE SKIN
3 drops each rose and lavender
in 30ml (1fl oz/6 tsps) olive oil

THE LEGS

FOR VARICOSE VEINS
2 drops each cypress, lime and marigold
in 30ml (1fl oz/6 tsps) sweet almond oil

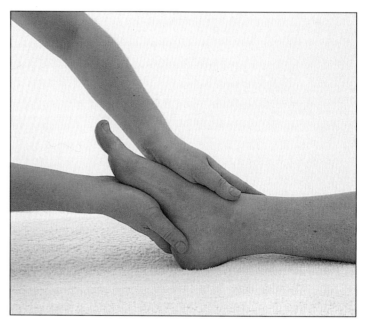

(Above) Reward your feet for all their hard work with a reviving essential oil massage.

FOR CELLULITE
4 drops each lavender, juniper and rosemary
in 60ml (1fl oz/6 tsps)of sesame oil

FOR STRETCH MARKS
3 drops lavender and 2 drops each frankincense and
sandalwood in 30ml (1fl oz/6 tsps) sesame oil

FOR FLUID RETENTION
3 drops cypress and 2 drops each geranium and sage
in 30ml (1fl oz/6 tsps) sweet almond oil

THE ARMS

FOR SLACK SKIN ON UPPER ARMS
2 drops each geranium, lemongrass and marjoram
in 30ml (1fl oz/6 tsps) sesame oil

FOR DRY SKIN ON ELBOWS
2 drops each chamomile, jasmine and sandalwood
in 30ml (1fl oz/6 tsps) olive oil

THE HANDS

FOR NAILS
3 drops each bay and sandalwood
in 30ml (1fl oz/6 tsps) sweet almond oil

FOR SKIN
2 drops each lavender, geranium and chamomile
in 30ml (1fl oz/6 tsps) sweet almond oil

THE BACK

FOR SPOTS AND OILINESS
2 drops each chamomile, bergamot and basil in 30ml
(1fl oz/6 tsps) safflower oil

THE BODY

FOR SCARS
3 drops lavender and 2 drops neroli
in 15ml (0.5fl oz/3 tsps) wheatgerm oil

FOR EXCESS PERSPIRATION
3 drops citronella and 2 drops each lemongrass and
bergamot in 30ml (1fl oz/6 tsps) sunflower oil

FOR ENERGY
2 drops each peppermint, rosemary and lemongrass
in 60ml (2fl oz/12 tsps) sweet almond oil

FOR RELAXATION
7 drops each jasmine and neroli
in 60ml (2fl oz/12 tsps)sweet almond oil

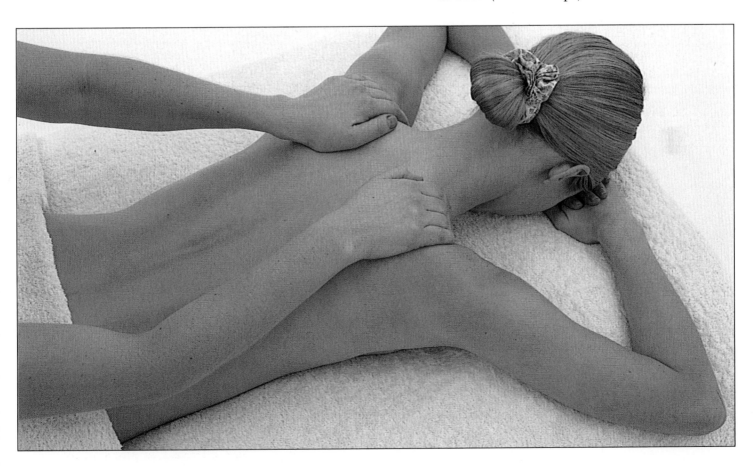

(Above) Chamomile, bergamot and basil are ideal for a blemished back.

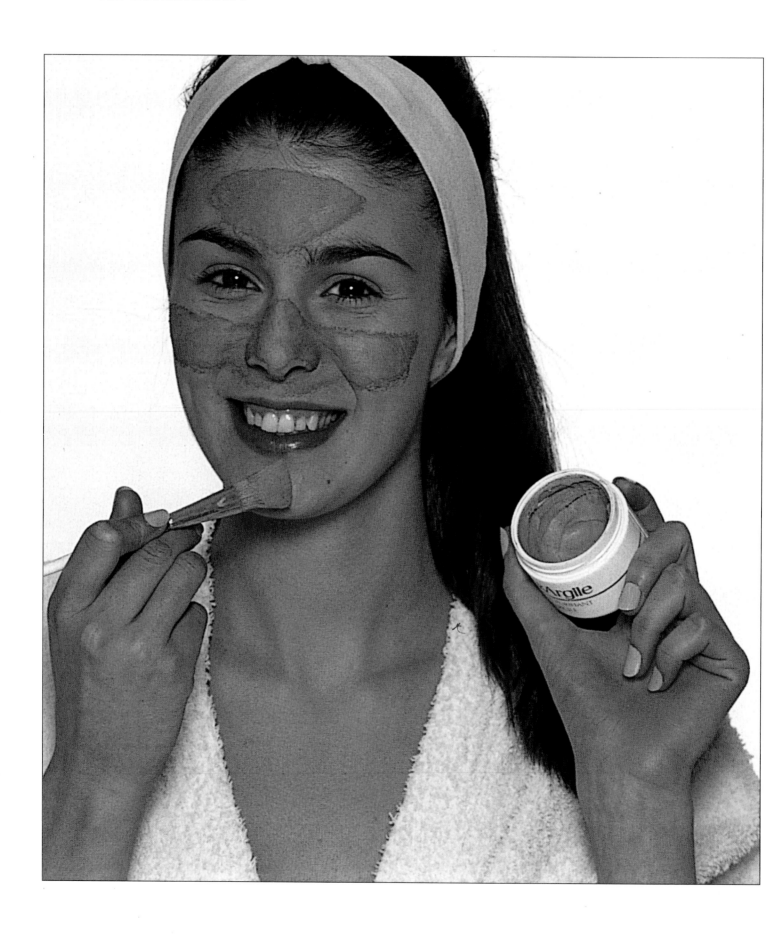

Essential Oils for the Face

A healthy, glowing complexion is the one thing most women say is the sign of true beauty. And so they spend more on skincare than on any other beauty products. Consequently, the cosmetics industry has created thousands of potions for the face alone – cleansers, toners, moisturisers, exfoliators, masks, eye creams and gels, neck creams, anti-ageing serums, sun and anti-pollution protectors...

In all honesty, all you really need is the right essential oil. They can be used to do every one of these jobs, and the wide range of their properties means they can do it in the best possible way to suit your skin's needs.

If you create your own essential-oil beauty products you know exactly what is in them, they are custom-blended, extremely effective, aromatically fragranced, and since you're not paying for expensive advertising campaigns or fancy packaging, they are ridiculously cheap.

THE BEST BEAUTY PRODUCTS

You can use essential oils to make products for facial moisturising, anti-ageing treatments, exfoliating, toning and deep cleansing – in other words, for your complete beauty routine. And you can design each product to treat every skin type or problem, from mature or dry complexions, to open pores or acne. When using essential-oil beauty products on the face, be careful to avoid the eyes and the inside of the mouth and nose as these areas are sensitive and essential oils are potent.

Since essential oils treat mind and mood as much as purely physical complaints, make sure you use the best combination of oils to make you feel good and look good. For instance, if you have dry skin you could treat it with rose and lavender oils on a day when you are tense, so you soothe mental worries and your complexion in one go; or if you are tired at the end of a hard day, use geranium and neroli oils to rejuvenate your spirits and looks at the same time.

(Left) Try out different face mask recipes to find one that suits you.

Although all essential oils are absorbed by skin more effectively than the ingredients of most cosmetic face creams, some essential oils are better for the fragile facial skin than others. This is because the face is exposed to climate, pollutants and sunlight all day, unlike body skin. So the soothing, healing, rejuvenating essential oils will have a much more noticeable effect on facial skin than any other oils. To help guide you, here is a list of the most useful oils for the face.

Best Aromatic Oils

geranium

jasmine

lavender

neroli

rose

violet

ylang-ylang

•

Best Therapeutic Oils

chamomile

(rashes, itchiness)

•

juniper

(acne, oiliness)

•

lemongrass

(open pores)

•

mandarin

(scars, slack skin)

•

marigold

(over dry, sensitive)

•

mimosa

(dull complexions)

•

orange

(wrinkles, sallowness)

ESSENTIAL CLEANSERS

Some women don't think their faces are clean until they have splashed them with water while others prefer to use a cotton ball soaked in cream cleansing-lotion. However, no matter which routine you follow, it is easy to add benefits from essential oils. And since essential oils penetrate skin quickly and easily, they deep-cleanse pores and treat problems simultaneously. The best oils to cleanse gently and soothe skin on a daily basis are:

For dry/mature skin: neroli
For normal/combination: skin rose
For oily/blemished skin: lavender

THE WATER RINSE

If you wash with soap and water, add two drops of essential oil to a basin of warm water for the final face rinse. Gently stir with your fingers to disperse the oil droplets before splashing and patting the water on your face. If you have time, leave the water to air-dry rather than using a towel so the essential oils are left as a film on the skin's surface.

The Oil Slick

If you usually use a light, oil-based lotion to remove make-up and cleanse your face, replace it with three drops of essential oil added to 30ml (1fl oz/6 tsps) of sweet almond oil. Store the mix in a dark glass bottle and shake well before pouring some into the palm of your hand and using your fingertips to massage it into skin. Gently wipe it off with a damp cotton-wool pad and if any stubborn patches of make-up remain, remove them by dipping a cotton-wool ball directly into the oil mix and gently wiping across skin.

The Cream Clean

If you like to use a cream cleanser on your face, you may add the aroma and benefits of essential oils to your usual cosmetic product. Buy the simplest, fragrance-free cleansing-cream you can find and add four drops of essential oil for every 50ml (1.7fl oz/10 tsps) of product in the jar. Mix the essential oil into the cleanser using a sterile spatula or teaspoon handle, replace the lid and leave it for three days. Stir the mixture once a day before you begin to use it. Apply it and remove as you normally would.

However, if you notice that the formulation changes in texture during this three-day period, becoming thicker, thinner or lumpy, throw it away. Occasionally the emulsion of a particular brand of cream becomes unstable if you add extra ingredients and it may eventually lead to bacterial contamination.

The Smooth Option

For truly polished skin, free of dull, dead, flaky surface cells, use a gentle essential-oil exfoliator twice a week. Mix three drops of essential oil with 30ml (1fl oz/6 tsps) sweet almond oil and slowly add equal amounts of finely ground oatmeal and coarse dessicated coconut until you have a thick paste. Rub the paste in small circular movements all over damp skin, particularly around the forehead, nose, chin and neck, then leave for a few minutes before rinsing off with tepid water. Pat skin dry and moisturise immediately.

Cleanser Trouble Spots

To make essential oils even more effective, use the same treatment throughout your entire beauty routine. For instance, if you have a very oily complexion, treat the problem by adding your favourite-smelling anti-grease essential oils to your cleanser, toner and moisturiser. Then you can boost your treatment using individual oils in weekly exfoliators, masks or steam facials, to treat particular skin trouble spots.

You may also mix a facial moisturiser for dry areas and one for oily patches, or do the same with cleansers or face masks, and apply each type just where it is needed. The more you look to your own, personal skin problems and treat them individually, the more your complexion will benefit which is something you can never afford to do with conventional beauty products.

If you want to customise your cleansers, turn to the recipes suggested for facial moisturiser (see page 88) and use those particular essential oil combinations so that the various stages of your skincare routine are in unison with each other.

ESSENTIAL MOISTURISERS

Facial moisturisers that use essential oils give you the chance to create amazingly personal skincare products. You can mix small amounts so the ingredients are always fresh without any wastage; you can mix several different combinations for different parts of your face and apply them just where needed; and since essential oils are so fine and have a natural affinity with skin, they penetrate better than many ingredients found in more traditional face creams.

When to Use Them

Like any moisturiser, they should be applied morning and night to well-cleansed skin. However, you can use a richer carrier oil and more moisturising essential oils for a night treatment if you wish and create a lighter formulation for summer than in winter. Some of the treatment essential-oil combinations may not smell as good as some of the single oils, such as the orange-blossom-scented neroli, so you can always apply a moisturiser for pleasure and aroma in the morning and save the treatment products for night time.

How to Use Them

The best way to apply a facial moisturiser is sparingly. Too much leaves skin looking greasy and shiny and may cause blackheads or other excess oil problems. Massage is the best way to make sure the oils soak in, as the warmth of skin on skin and the rubbing action both speed up absorption. Spend three minutes minimum gently smoothing the moisturiser all over your face, using fingertips in an upwards direction and in circles from the inner to outer corners of the eyes. Better still, use the facial self-massage (see page 124) once a day to relax and help restore tone to skin.

Remember to mix only enough to last for a few days so there is no risk of contamination. Always store your moisturisers in airtight, dark glass bottles and shake them well before application. The ideal recipe should be:

FOR FACIAL MOISTURISERS
5 drops essential oil in 30ml (1fl oz/6 tsps)
carrier oil plus 1 tsp wheatgerm oil
– OR –
the contents of a vitamin E capsule.

How to Blend Them
All facial moisturisers should contain essential oils, carrier oil to dilute, and either wheatgerm oil or vitamin E. The latter act as a natural preservative, and as they are also both excellent anti-oxidants they add an extra treatment benefit to your skincare.

The latest theories on skin damage and ageing claim that cells degenerate when external irritants like sunlight, pollution or cigarette smoke cause them to oxidise – a similar process to when an apple rots or metal rusts. Research shows that anti-oxidants stop this degeneration and help compensate for damage caused on a daily basis by skin irritants.

In fact, most cosmetic face-creams now contain vitamins C, E and A, the best anti-oxidants to help prevent skin ageing. So by adding wheatgerm, which contains a high amount of vitamin E, or pure vitamin E, by pricking a capsule with a pin and squeezing out the contents, you are adding an anti-ageing ingredient to every facial moisturiser you mix.

The other bonus is that carrier oils, used to dilute the essential oils, are excellent moisturisers in themselves. Remember it is oil on the skin's surface, and not a secret wet ingredient, that makes a good moisturiser. The oils stops the water found naturally in the body from evaporating into the air.

The best carrier oils for the face are fine, light emollients. Some of the heavier oils are too rich and sit on facial skin for hours making the complexion shiny.

Moisturiser Trouble Spots
To make your own facial moisturiser recipes, use the charts to check essential oils' properties (see page 50).

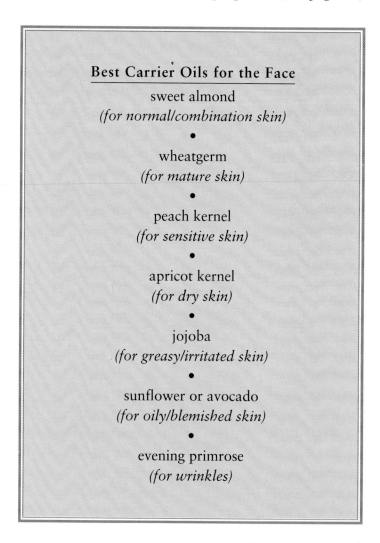

Best Carrier Oils for the Face

sweet almond
(for normal/combination skin)

•

wheatgerm
(for mature skin)

•

peach kernel
(for sensitive skin)

•

apricot kernel
(for dry skin)

•

jojoba
(for greasy/irritated skin)

•

sunflower or avocado
(for oily/blemished skin)

•

evening primrose
(for wrinkles)

Check that your choice of oils will mix well (see page 46). You may also try a blotting paper sniff test (see page 14) to make sure the final aromatic combination pleases your nose.

RICH FACIAL MOISTURISERS

FOR MATURE SKIN
3 drops neroli and 2 drops galbanum
in 30ml (1fl oz/6 tsps) wheatgerm oil
– OR –
2 drops each rose and frankincense
in 30ml (1fl oz/6 tsps) evening primrose oil
plus 1 vitamin E capsule

FOR DRY SKIN
2 drops violet and 3 drops rose in 30ml (1fl oz/6 tsps)
apricot kernel oil plus 1 vitamin E capsule
– OR –
2 drops each neroli, mimosa and rose
in 30ml (1fl oz/6 tsps) wheatgerm oil

FOR THREAD VEINS
3 drops rose and 2 drops chamomile in 30ml
(1fl oz/6 tsps) peach oil plus 1 tsp wheatgerm oil
– OR –
3 drops orange and 1 drop each lemon and lime in
30ml (1fl oz/6 tsps) peach oil plus 1 tsp wheatgerm oil

TO TREAT RASHES, ITCHINESS
2 drops chamomile and 3 drops lavender in
30ml (1fl oz/6 tsps) peach oil plus 1 vitamin E capsule
– OR –
1 drop each marigold and yarrow and 3 drops of
sandalwood in 30ml (1fl oz/6 tsps) jojoba oil
plus 1 tsp wheatgerm oil

TO FIRM SKIN
3 drops frankincense and 2 drops mandarin in
30ml (1fl oz/6 tsps) wheatgerm oil
– OR –
2 drops each rose and lavender and 1 drop neroli
in 30ml (1fl oz/6 tsps) wheatgerm oil

TO IMPROVE TEXTURE
3 drops violet and 2 drops lemongrass in
30ml (1fl oz/6 tsps) evening primrose oil
plus 1 vitamin E capsule
– OR –
2 drops each sandalwood and geranium and 1 drop
rose in 30ml (1fl oz/6 tsps) wheatgerm oil

FOR NIGHT TIME
2 drops each frankincense and myrrh in
30ml (1fl oz/6 tsps) wheatgerm oil

LIGHT MOISTURISERS

FOR OILY SKIN
2 drops each juniper and cedarwood in 30ml
(1fl oz/6 tsps) sunflower oil plus 1 vitamin E capsule
– OR –
2 drops each geranium and lavender and 1 drop
cypress in 30ml (1fl oz/6 tsps) of sunflower oil
plus 1 vitamin E capsule

FOR COMBINATION SKIN
2 drops each lemongrass and rosemary in
30ml (1fl oz/6 tsps) sweet almond oil
plus 1 vitamin E capsule
– OR –
1 drop petitgrain and 2 drops each rose and
lavender in 30ml (1fl oz/6 tsps) sweet almond oil
plus 1 vitamin E capsule

FOR SENSITIVE SKIN
2 drops marigold and 3 drops rosemary in
30ml (1fl oz/6 tsps) peach oil
plus 1 tsp wheatgerm oil
– OR –
2 drops each chamomile and jasmine and 1 drop
sandalwood in 30ml (1fl oz/6 tsps) jojoba oil
plus 1 vitamin E capsule

TO TREAT SALLOWNESS
3 drops orange and 2 drops rosemary in 30ml (1fl oz/6 tsps) jojoba oil plus 1 tsp wheatgerm oil
– OR –
2 drops each lavender and ylang-ylang and 1 drop geranium in 30ml (1fl oz/6 tsps) sunflower oil plus 1 vitamin E capsule

---

TO TREAT ACNE
3 drops bergamot and 2 drops chamomile in 30ml (1fl oz/6 tsps) sunflower oil plus 1 vitamin E capsule
– OR –
2 drops each lavender and mint and 1 drop lemon in 30ml (1fl oz/6 tsps) sunflower oil plus 1 vitamin E capsule

---

TO CLEAR BLACKHEADS
2 drops each tea tree and eucalyptus in 30ml (1fl oz/6 tsps) avocado oil plus 1 vitamin E capsule
– OR –
2 drops each lavender and geranium and 1 drop lemon in 30ml (1fl oz/6 tsps) sunflower oil plus 1 vitamin E capsule

---

FOR DAY TIME
2 drops violet and 3 drops rose in 30ml (1fl oz/6 tsps) sweet almond oil plus 1 vitamin E capsule

ESSENTIAL FACE MASKS

Mixing your own essential-oil face pack takes five minutes, using simple ingredients you should have in your kitchen, is a lot of fun and gives you a very effective product. The other bonus is that you only make enough for a single application so there is no waste and you can try different combinations as often as you want. Not only that, but by adding the mask ingredient, or the paste that has the drawing effect on skin, you also help hold the essential oils in place on the

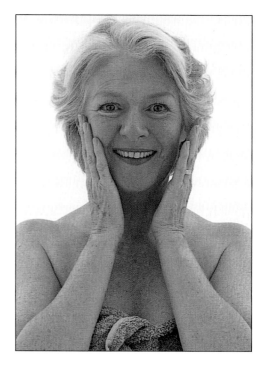

(Left) Dry or mature skin benefits from the regenerative powers of frankincense.

(Below) Avoid applying your face mask too close to eyes, nostrils and lips.

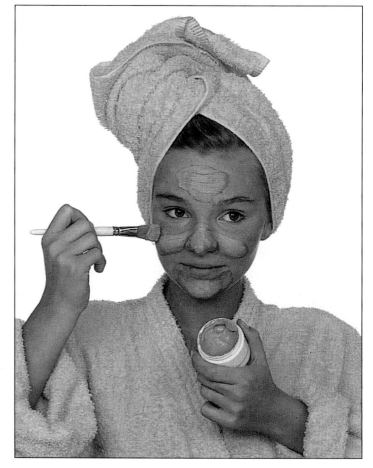

skin's surface so they're absorbed, rather than evaporating into the air, and are even more beneficial.

The best oils to fix to the skin surface for a deep facial treatment are:

For mature/dry skin: frankincense
For normal/combination skin: jasmine
For oily/blemished skin: geranium

When to Use Them

Face masks should be used as occasional cleansing or nourishing treatments to improve your complexion during times of stress, ill health, climatic or hormonal changes. If you overuse them they make skin drier or oilier by overstimulating it.

A deep-cleansing face mask should be used no more than once a week and a moisturising pack at most twice a week. It is best to use them at night and, since you have to lie back and rest while the mask does its work, include a relaxing or energising aromatic oil in the recipe to work on your mind at the same time.

How to Use Them

As soon as you have mixed up an essential-oil face mask, apply it to well-cleansed skin by smoothing it evenly on in upward strokes. Avoid the eye area, nostrils and lips, as skin here is very sensitive, but apply it to the neck right down to the collarbone. Then relax for 10-15 minutes until the mask has dried.

For a deep-cleansing facial, use your fingertips to rub the dried mask off your skin so you exfoliate it at the same time, then wash any residue off. For a moisturising facial, rinse the mask off with warm water until skin is clean.

How to Blend Them

Only mix enough mask for one application: it won't keep for more than an hour or two. Any leftovers can be spread on elbows, knees or upper back. To mix an essential-oil mask, place all ingredients in a small bowl and stir well with a teaspoon. You will need a powdery ingredient to give the right paste-like consistency. The best are:

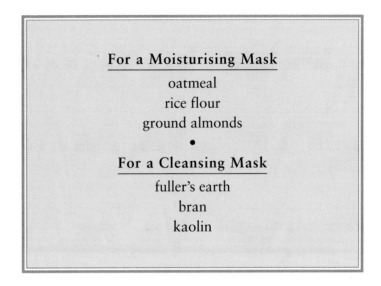

For a Moisturising Mask
oatmeal
rice flour
ground almonds

•

For a Cleansing Mask
fuller's earth
bran
kaolin

The finer the powdery ingredient the more the mask will tighten and draw out grime from the skin, so put the oatmeal, bran or almonds in a food processor and blend them if they are too coarse. You can make any moisturising mask more effective by adding a teaspoon of warm, melted honey. A cleansing mask will be more drawing if you heat it before application. Put the prepared paste in a screw-top glass jar and stand it in a container of just-boiled water for a few minutes until it has warmed through. The ideal recipe should be:

FOR FACE MASKS

Moisturising

6 drops essential oil in 30ml (1fl oz/6 tsps) carrier oil mixed with enough powdery ingredient to make a sticky, thick paste

Cleansing

6 drops essential oil in 30ml (1fl oz/6 tsps) hot water mixed with enough powdery ingredient to make a smooth, thick paste

MASKS FOR TROUBLE SPOTS

You can easily make masks using a facial moisturiser-oil mix that you already have (see recipes on page 88). Just add enough powdery ingredient to make a paste. Or you can use a single oil that is particularly suited to skincare (see best aromatic/therapeutic oils, page 50) and particularly suits your own sense of smell.

Remember also that you can apply several different masks in patches: a moisturising one over dry cheeks, an oil-control mix for nose and chin and a firming mix for the jaw and neck, for instance. After removing the mask, you may like to apply a little massage oil to the skin, or a blend of 15 drops rose oil in 30 ml (1fl oz/6 tsps) jojoba. Here are some recipes for the most common types of mask so you can perfect mixing them before you go on to experiment alone.

BASIC FACE MASKS

Moisturising mask
2 drops each frankincense, rose, neroli in 30ml (1fl oz/6 tsps) apricot oil with 1 tsp warmed, melted, clear honey, mixed with enough finely ground almond to make a soft paste

Deep cleansing mask
2 drops geranium, 3 drops lavender and 1 drop lemon in 30ml (1fl oz/6 tsps) hot water, mixed with enough kaolin to make a smooth paste

Relaxing mask
2 drops each violet, lavender and neroli in 30 ml (1fl oz/6 tsps) sweet almond oil, with enough oatmeal to make a smooth paste

Energising mask
2 drops each ylang-ylang, petitgrain and lemon in 30ml (1fl oz/6 tsps) iced water, with enough ground almond to make a smooth paste

Anti-ageing mask
2 drops each neroli, mandarin and orange in 30ml (1fl oz/6 tsps) evening primrose oil with 1 tsp of warmed, melted clear honey, mixed with enough ground almond to make a smooth paste

ESSENTIAL STEAM FACIALS

There is one other remarkably effective way to use essential oils in your beauty routine. Simply add them to a steam facial. There is double benefit in this method. The steam opens pores and warms skin, so essential oils are absorbed more rapidly. It also makes the oils themselves more volatile, so they evaporate faster and are even more aromatic than usual. The steam facial is also deeply relaxing, quick and non-messy.

However, since it is so effective, some essential oils are too potent to be directly inhaled in such a small space and absorbed with steam in this way, especially as they enter the nasal passages and can irritate eyes. Steam facials are not recommended for anyone with a history of asthma or respiratory complaints. Do not use the oils listed on the following page, as they have an irritating effect when inhaled.

When to Use a Steam Facial
Steam facials should be used to deep-cleanse or deep-moisturise skin once a week at most, in place of a face mask. They are particularly effective when skin is dull, dehydrated, spotty or greasy, as they act as an instant beautifier.

However, don't use them just before you plan to go out as the heat and steam can leave a high colour on the cheeks and make skin look shiny for a couple of hours afterwards. Since they are so relaxing it is best to use them before going to bed. Also, any moisturiser you apply afterwards will get to work on warmed, softened skin and immediately become an extra beneficial night cream.

Oils Not Recommended for Steam Facials

basil	citronella
laurel	tea tree
bay	fennel
pine	thyme
birch	ginger
clary sage	valerian
camphor	juniper
tarragon	

How to use them

Wearing an off-the-shoulder top, cleanse the skin thoroughly. Then boil some water. Pour the required amount into a large, heat-retaining bowl and place it on a table. Make sure it is the right height so you can sit comfortably and bend forwards over the bowl. Have a large towel ready to drape over your head and trap the steam. Then add your chosen essential oils drop by drop onto the surface of the water.

Stay under the towel with your eyes closed until the steam cools then add more boiling water to the bowl to evaporate off any remaining essential oils. Afterwards, gently pat your face dry and immediately apply a moisturiser to trap the extra steamy water in your skin.

FOR STEAM FACIALS
Add 5 drops essential oil
to 1 litre (2 pints) boiling water

Steam Facial Trouble Spots

It is best to use a maximum of two different essential oils in a steam facial because they become so aromatic with the heat that any more are invariably overpowering. However, the right combination will treat almost any problem of both the skin and psyche. Here is a selection of recipes for you to try before you start creating your own concoctions:

DEEP CLEANSING FACIAL

FOR DRY SKIN
2 drops lavender and 3 drops of violet

FOR NORMAL / COMBINATION SKIN
2 drops mimosa and 3 drops geranium

FOR OILY / BLEMISHED SKIN
3 drops juniper and 2 drops bergamot

FOR MATURE SKIN
3 drops frankincense and 2 drops galbanum

DEEP MOISTURISING FACIAL

FOR DRY SKIN
2 drops chamomile and 3 drops of jasmine

FOR NORMAL / COMBINATION SKIN
2 drops rose and 3 drops sandalwood

FOR OILY / BLEMISHED SKIN
2 drops chamomile and 3 drops geranium

FOR MATURE SKIN
2 drops of neroli and 3 drops rose

RELAXING FACIAL

2 drops of ylang-ylang and 3 drops jasmine

INVIGORATING FACIAL

2 drops of peppermint and 3 drops lavender

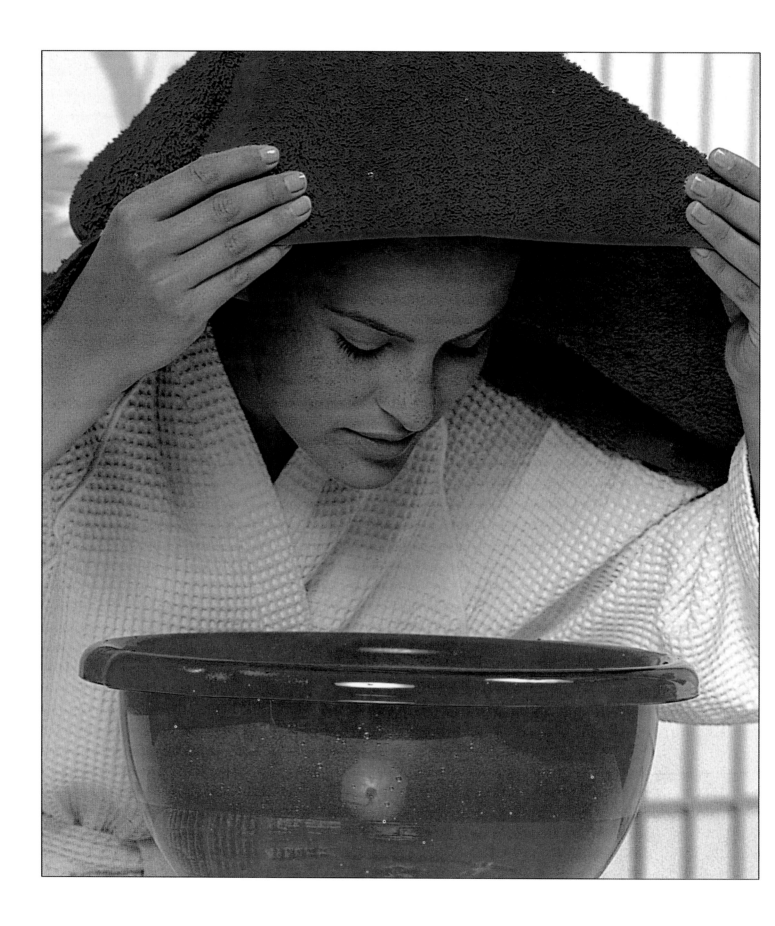

INHALING ESSENTIAL OILS

When you breathe in the aroma of an essential oil it affects you in many ways.
Firstly, the smell itself is instantly recorded in the limbic area of the brain, where we
also store memories and emotions. This is why a whiff of antiseptic can
make you think of being in hospital and feel afraid, if this is what your memory of
antiseptics is. Or the smell of lavender makes you think of having a cuddle with your
grandmother, if she used it as a perfume, and feeling safe and happy.
This is the reason why you either love or hate a particular smell,
and why your sense of smell is such a personal thing.

Secondly, the miniscule chemical elements that make up each molecule of an essential
oil are absorbed through the nasal membranes and can, for instance, relax
the nervous system, make you feel more alert, or change your mood. Although
researchers still don't understand how this happens, they have physical
proof that it does. They know, for example, that inhaling a relaxing smell causes
an immediate reduction in blood pressure and slows the heart beat.

Both of these things tell us that inhaling essential oils is a quick, simple and effective
way of enjoying their therapeutic benefits. If you use aromatherapy on a daily
basis, it is also a good way to test and strengthen your sense of smell and
improve your health and well-being. And, anyone who
sets foot in your home will benefit, too.

Here is a guide to how to prepare and use essential oils for inhalation,
with some of the best essential oil combinations for each method.

(Left) Stress-related problems respond quickly to aromatic inhalations.

95

INHALATION

Best method:

Inhaling the oils with warm steam in a small space means you get maximum benefits in minimum time. It is ideal for treating coughs or colds, or for treating your skin to a steam facial (see page 92). The best method is to place 1 litre (2 pints) of boiling water in a heat-retaining bowl, and add five drops of essential oil to the surface of the water. Bend forwards over the bowl and drape a large towel over your head to trap the evaporating oils and steam. Inhale the vapours for a few minutes, then add a little more boiling water to evaporate off any remaining essential oil.

You may also inhale undiluted essential oils from a tissue or handkerchief, but only in moderation. Two drops of oil tipped directly onto the fabric is enough to last for several hours. Place it on your pillow at night or in your breast pocket or bra during the day.

Best Oils for Inhalation

chamomile
(for sleeplessness)

•

eucalyptus
(for chest/nasal congestion)

•

frankincense
(depression, anxiety)

•

myrrh
(for sore throat, coughs)

•

peppermint
(for energy, concentration)

ROOM VAPORISERS

Best method:

You can buy essential-oil burners which have a saucer

Best Oils for Room Vapourisers

bergamot
(uplifting, refreshing, deodorising)

•

eucalyptus
(for chest/nasal congestion, mental alertness)

•

geranium
(energising yet relaxing)

•

jasmine
(for euphoria, confidence, dinner parties)

•

lavender
(for tension, nerves, tiredness)

•

mandarin
(for sleeplessness, soothing, calming)

•

neroli
(calming, soothing, sensual)

•

peppermint
(for energy, alertness)

•

sandalwood
(relaxing, mellowing, romantic)

•

ylang-ylang
(hypnotic, sensual, uplifting)

fixed above a stand which holds a candle. Fill the saucer with hot water, add up to eight drops of essential oil, and light the candle to keep the water hot enough to make the oil evaporate. They scent a room quickly and only need to be placed on a steady, safe surface out of the reach of children or pets. Top up with water and oil every three to four hours.

You can make your own version by standing a saucer of hot water on top of a central-heating radiator, although this does not evaporate the oils as speedily as the heat of a candle.

You can also buy small metal or compressed card rings, which sit on top of an ordinary light bulb and gently warm the four or five drops of essential oil placed on them. They scent a room quickly and almost as potently as the burners.

Electronic diffusers (known as nebulisers) are useful since essential oils can be used without being heated and thus altered.

It is best to use only single essential oils to scent a room, as combinations of more than one don't keep their individual aromas particularly well. However, you can change oils every day if you wish, so there is plenty of variation.

ROOM SPRAYS

Best method:
For a natural, non-aerosol and highly aromatic air-freshener, add ten drops of essential oil to half a litre (one pint) of water in a pump-action, spray bottle (the kind used for watering houseplants). Shake the mixture well before pumping four or five sprays into the air to deodorise, freshen and scent a room.

POT POURRI

Best method:
Make your own pot pourri by mixing together dried leaves, flowers and herbs from your garden (geranium, rose, lavender, pinks, cornflowers, citrus blossoms, etc) with spices (cinnamon sticks, cloves, nutmeg, allspice), a little talcum powder and favourite essential oils. The basic mix should contain six cups of dried plants, two

---

Best Oils for Freshening

lavender
(to kill airborne germs in the house)

•

lemon
(air freshener for the toilet)

•

peppermint
(to remove the stale smell of cigarette smoke)

•

Best Combinations

3 drops each pine, rosemary and lavender
(disinfecting, for bathrooms, rubbish bins, damp or mould)

•

5 drops each lemon and lime
(deodorising, for wardrobes, cupboards, bathrooms, cooking smells)

---

tablespoons of talc and 12 drops of essential oils.

Leave it in an airtight container, shaking and inverting it daily for a fortnight until the aromas have been absorbed by the talc and dried materials. Then place it in an open bowl or jar to fragrance a room. Refresh it when needed by adding a few more drops of essential oils.

WOOD FIRES

Since heat makes essential oils more potent, pour a maximum of 12 drops on three pieces of wood about 15 minutes before lighting the fire. It will warm and scent your room simultaneously. If you don't have an open fire, a similar effect can be achieved by dropping your favourite essence onto a radiator.

Best Oils for Wood Fires

geranium	patchouli
neroli	lemon
jasmine	rose
orange	lime
lavender	sandalwood

Best Combinations

FOR WINTER

4 drops each ginger, orange and sandalwood

FOR SUMMER

4 drops each bergamot, geranium, lavender

USING OILS IN THE HOME

Using essential oils around your home does more than get rid of bad smells and bad tempers. Many oils have powerful disinfectant properties that kill germs and improve hygiene more effectively than many household cleansers. There's an added bonus too: the oils really are natural and don't need any environmentally damaging chemical additives to help them clean properly.

For most cleansing jobs you need only a few drops of essential oil, so you will find they are amazingly economical and long-lasting. And in some cases, it is best to use the smallest quantity of oils possible, so they disinfect without leaving a noticeable aroma.

Here are some suggestions of ways to use oils to cleanse, protect and purify your home, plus the best oils to do the job.

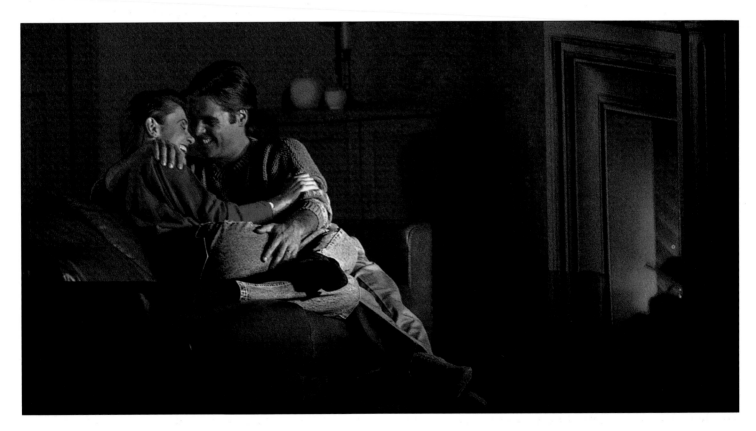

(Above) Set the scene with drops of fresh or spicy oils on a wood fire.

> ### Best Household Oils
>
> | | |
> |---|---|
> | lavender | geranium |
> | bergamot | peppermint |
> | myrrh | lime |
> | eucalyptus | pine |
> | orange | mandarin |
> | cedarwood | sandalwood |

AIR PURIFIER

Best method:

Not only can you make your whole house smell fresh, but you can also purify the air by adding essential oils to the dust bag of your vacuum cleaner. Place five drops of oil on a cotton-wool ball inside the cleaner, against the exit filter where air blows out of your machine. To refresh or change the fragrance, just replace it with a new cotton ball as often as you wish.

> ### Best Purifying Oils
>
> | | |
> |---|---|
> | bergamot | peppermint |
> | citronella | pine |
> | lavender | rosemary |
> | lemon | tea tree |

CLEANSERS

Best method:

To wipe kitchen surfaces and chopping boards and to wash floors, add eight drops of essential oil to a small bucket of warm water, wring out a cloth.

To clean basins, toilets, baths, and sinks, put three drops of essential oil on a damp cloth.

To sterilise dishes and cutlery, add two drops of essential oil to the washing-up water.

To rinse clothes, add three drops of essential oil to the final rinsing water.

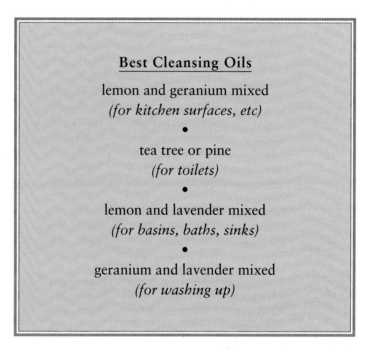

> ### Best Cleansing Oils
>
> lemon and geranium mixed
> *(for kitchen surfaces, etc)*
>
> •
>
> tea tree or pine
> *(for toilets)*
>
> •
>
> lemon and lavender mixed
> *(for basins, baths, sinks)*
>
> •
>
> geranium and lavender mixed
> *(for washing up)*

DEODORISERS

Best method:

To disinfect the air in a sickroom, burn oils as already described, in a vaporizer.

To deodorise and neutralise odours, put four drops of essential oil on a cotton-wool ball and place it in a wardrobe, laundry basket, rubbish bin, shoe rack, etc.

For persistent underarm odour, place two drops of essential oil on the inside, underarm seams of shirts, jackets or jumpers.

For smelly shoes, rub four drops of essential oil into the insoles with a tissue.

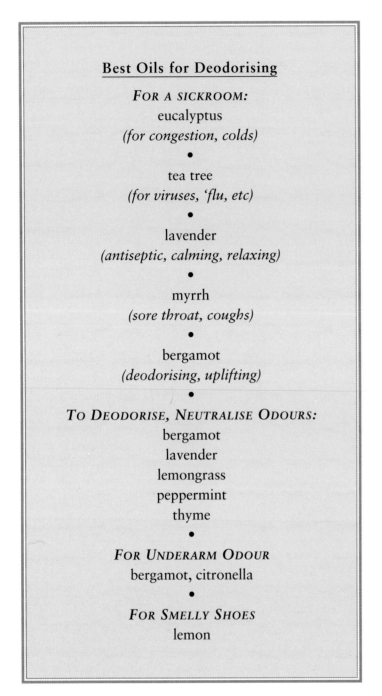

Best Oils for Deodorising

FOR A SICKROOM:
eucalyptus
(for congestion, colds)

•

tea tree
(for viruses, 'flu, etc)

•

lavender
(antiseptic, calming, relaxing)

•

myrrh
(sore throat, coughs)

•

bergamot
(deodorising, uplifting)

•

TO DEODORISE, NEUTRALISE ODOURS:
bergamot
lavender
lemongrass
peppermint
thyme

•

FOR UNDERARM ODOUR
bergamot, citronella

•

FOR SMELLY SHOES
lemon

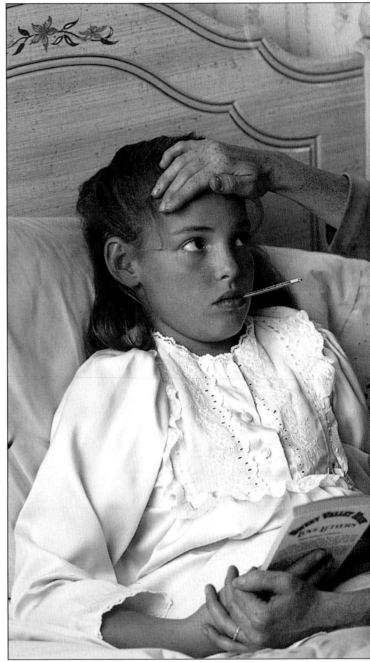

POULTICES

Best method:
This is an ideal way to use essential oils to relieve muscular pain and chest congestion. Add five drops of essential oil to 100ml (20fl oz/1 pint) of very hot water in saucepan, then cover it. Wearing rubber gloves, remove the lid and lay a folded cloth or flannel over the surface of the water to absorb oil. Squeeze out excess water and place it over the affected area until it has cooled to blood temperature. Reheat and repeat. Always test a poultice before applying to skin to ensure it isn't too hot.

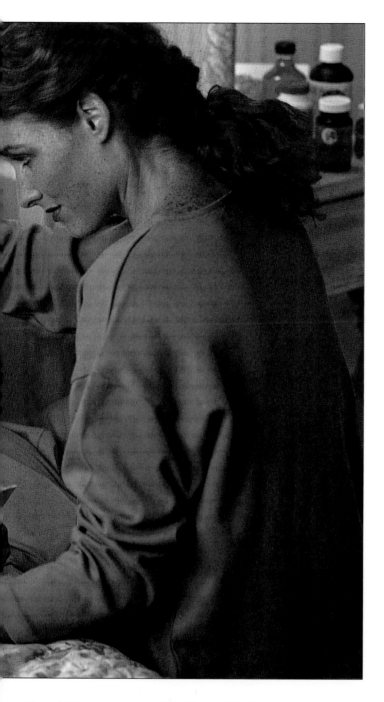

(Above) Vaporised essential oils quickly freshen and disinfect the air in a sickroom.

Use hot poultices for: backache, earache (one drop of oil on a damp cotton-wool ball), cramps, boils, aching feet, arthritis, rheumatism, tummy ache, stiff neck, muscular pain, sore throat or chest congestion.

Best Oils for Poultices

lavender, eucalyptus, petitgrain
(backache)

•

lavender
(earache)

•

ambrette, cypress, tarragon, juniper,
peppermint, clary sage
(cramps)

•

clary sage, galbanum, lemongrass,
tea tree, rosemary
(boils)

•

citronella, laurel, lemon, rosemary
(aching feet)

•

lime, myrrh, spruce
(arthritis)

•

angelica, lime, pine
(rheumatism)

•

angelica, cypress, fennel, ginger,
peppermint, tarragon
(tummy ache)

•

spruce, eucalyptus
(stiff neck)

•

ambrette, basil, eucalyptus, bay, camphor, ginger,
petitgrain, pine, marjoram, rosemary
(muscular pain)

•

angelica, myrrh, eucalyptus, sandalwood,
ginger, peppermint, pine, thyme
(sore throat, congestion)

COLD COMPRESSES

Best method:
This is an ideal way to use essential oils to help soothe inflammation or reduce fever. Follow the same procedure as for hot poultices (see above) but place the oils in 100ml (20 fl oz/1pt) cold water with six ice cubes, in a bowl.

Use cold compresses for: headaches, sprains, inflammation, fever, swollen bumps, burns, blistered, sore feet, rashes, measles, chicken pox, sunburn or a hangover.

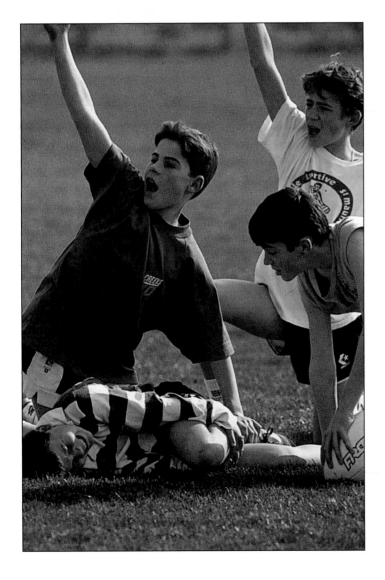

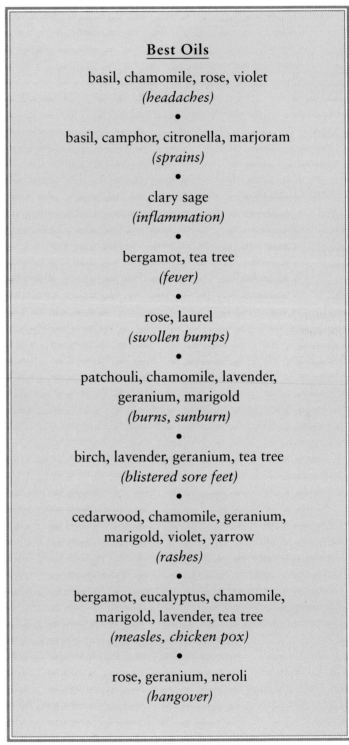

Best Oils

basil, chamomile, rose, violet
(headaches)

•

basil, camphor, citronella, marjoram
(sprains)

•

clary sage
(inflammation)

•

bergamot, tea tree
(fever)

•

rose, laurel
(swollen bumps)

•

patchouli, chamomile, lavender,
geranium, marigold
(burns, sunburn)

•

birch, lavender, geranium, tea tree
(blistered sore feet)

•

cedarwood, chamomile, geranium,
marigold, violet, yarrow
(rashes)

•

bergamot, eucalyptus, chamomile,
marigold, lavender, tea tree
(measles, chicken pox)

•

rose, geranium, neroli
(hangover)

(Left) Hot compresses ease muscular aches, while cold compresses soothe sprains.

INSECT REPELLENT

Best method:

Essential oils make excellent natural, fragrant, non-toxic insecticides which are kind to humans but absolutely repulsive to insects. Mix 15 drops of essential oils to 100ml (20fl oz/1 pint) water in a pump-action spray bottle and shake well before spritzing into the air to terrify flying insects. Or add five drops of essential oil to a damp cloth and wipe around wardrobes, shelves, drawers, window and door frames. Alternatively, apply oil drops directly to curtain hems to repel all airborne invaders.

A few drops of oil on your pillowcase or mattress will drive away droning mosquitoes. Or dilute six drops of the essential oil in 30ml (1fl oz/6 tsps) sunflower oil and rub it into any exposed skin before going to bed. It will also soothe the itchiness of any insect bites.

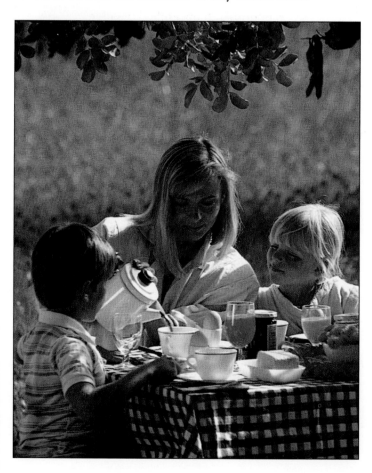

Best Oils

camphor
(moths)

•

citronella
(mosquitoes)

•

lemongrass
(most flying insects)

•

tea tree
(ants, fleas, most insects)

•

thyme
(most hopping/crawling insects)

•

Best Combinations

Dilute eight drops of tea tree
and seven drops of thyme in 30ml
(1fl oz/6 tsps) water in a spray bottle.
*(To get rid of ants or cockroaches spray
everywhere they might walk.)*

•

Dilute six drops of geranium, five drops
of lavender and four drops of tea tree in
30ml (1fl oz/6 tsps) of water in a spray bottle.
*(To rid a pet of fleas, spray into ruffled fur.
Avoid the eyes.)*

(Left) Citronella both deters marauding mosquitoes and soothes any bites.

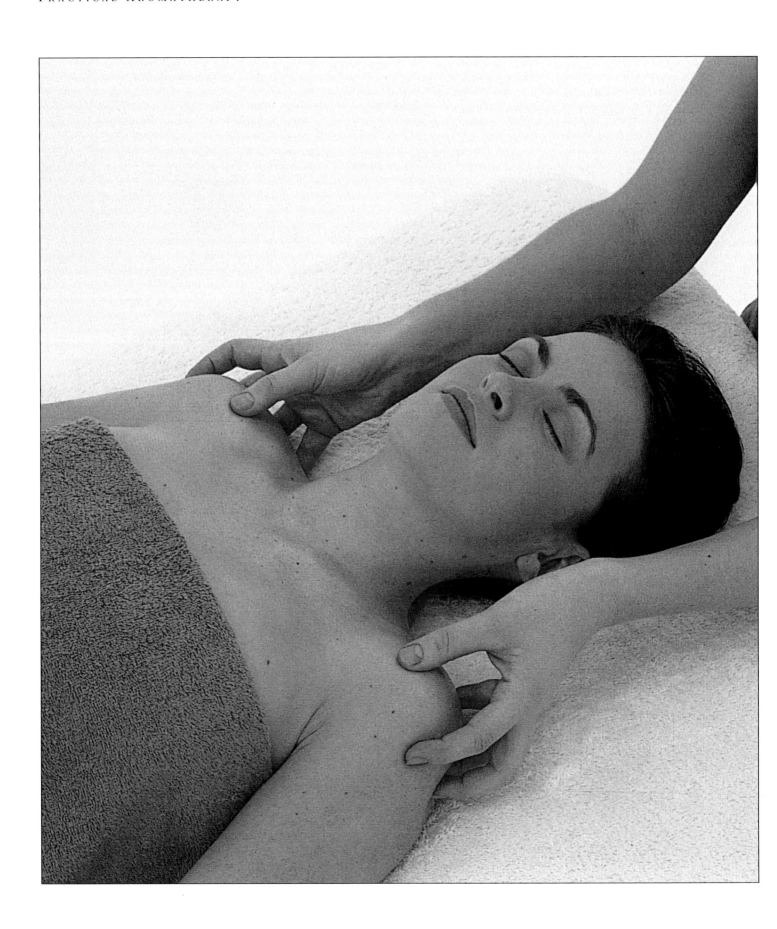

Using Essential Oils for Massage

Massage is the most common way of using essential oils, and it is the way they are used therapeutically in aromatherapy. Since it combines the two senses of touch and smell it has instant physical and mental benefits. The warm skin-on-skin friction from massage causes essential oils to be absorbed quicker and makes them more aromatic. And the same friction increases blood circulation, stimulates, relaxes muscles, lowers blood pressure and heart beat and makes you feel better than you could ever imagine.

Giving an aromatherapy massage is terribly simple. You don't have to be an expert, because the first rule of any type of massage is to trust your instincts. As you run your hands over the body, you should feel your way over the lumps, knotted muscles, tense or tender spots. Use the basic strokes but use your intuition as well, and make up the flow, rhythm and speed of the massage as you go along. If the recipient seems to like a particular stroke, keep doing it; if they wince, stop immediately and do something else. Try the same stroke quickly, slowly, firmly, lightly.

Prepare in advance. Read any instructions before you start, for if you balance an open book beside you and try to turn the pages with oily fingers it won't be a relaxing or pleasant experience for either of you.

Have a warm, comfortable environment and everything you need to hand, including the right essential oils. And then just to get on with it.

(Left) An aromatherapy massage is a deeply therapeutic experience.

HOW TO MASSAGE

The best way to learn to massage is to massage yourself. So four of the massages in this chapter, face/neck/scalp, energising top-to-toe, soothing foot and anti-age facial, are self-massages, while the last massage, relaxing back needs two people. While a do-it-yourself massage is deeply therapeutic, it is not quite as pleasurable as when someone else does it to you. And once you've mastered the basic routines single-handedly, it is quite easy to adapt them yourself and perform them on someone else.

Basic Strokes

Aromatherapy massage needs lots of long, slow strokes and short fast friction rubs to warm the oils and help move them into the skin. Keep your touch light over bony areas and the abdomen, but put more pressure on heavy muscles, such as the shoulders, buttocks and back. The main movements you will need to master are:

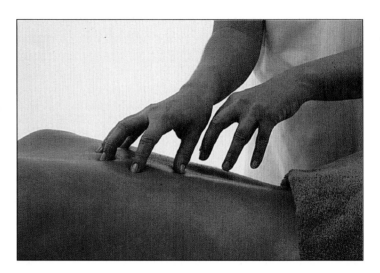

Raking

Pretend your fingertips are the ends of a rake. Keeping them bent but stiff at the joints, and with fingertips touching the skin, make firm, pulling movements back towards you. In this movement, you may choose to use both hands together, or one following the other in a repeated action.

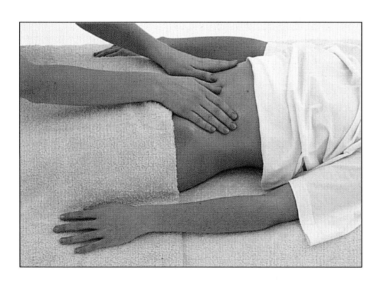

Stroking

This is the simplest massage movement, with both palms down and hands flat. You may do it with one hand following the other, as if you were stroking a cat. Or both hands parallel moving in unison in the same direction.

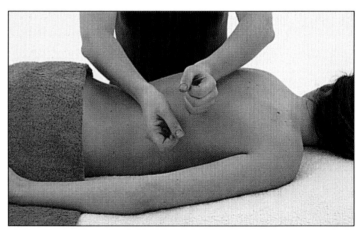

Pummelling

Making your hands into fists and keeping fingers relaxed, bounce them one after the other in a fast, drumming movement up and down on the body. You can do it with hands flat (i.e. pummelling with fingertips down), sideways (i.e. pummelling with thumbs up, little fingers down), or turned palm upwards (i.e. pummelling with backs of hands).

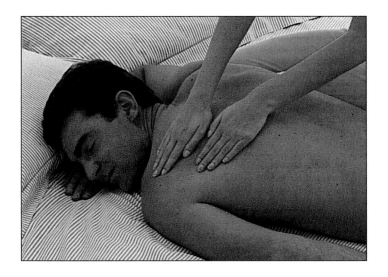

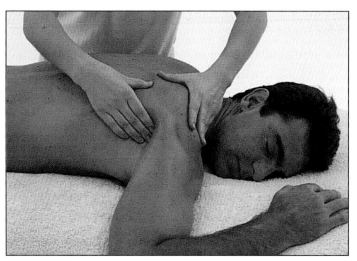

Friction Rub

With palms down and hands flat, move one up while the other moves down in a short, fast, sawing movement.

Kneading

Place your hands flat, fingers together with thumbs wide, then use your thumbs to push and pinch flesh up towards the fingers, moving them one after the other over the same area of flesh.

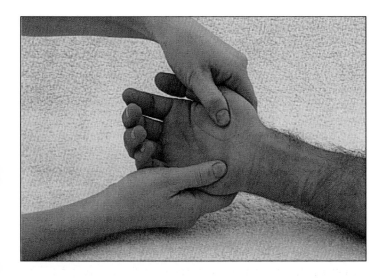

WHAT YOU WILL NEED

Apart from the right essential oil, an aromatherapy massage also needs a snug, warm room to make sure the evaporating oils are as aromatic as possible – and to stop you getting goose bumps. Peace and quiet are vital, so turn off the TV and take the phone off the hook.

For comfort, wear loose clothes that are easily removed and have lots of large towels to wrap yourself in or use as padding or pillows. Mix up just enough aromatherapy massage oil and, as glass is too slippery to hold when you have oily hands, place it in either a plastic bottle with a squirting top, or in a bowl that you can dip your fingers in.

Thumbing

Use the pad and side of your thumb to knead into flesh, stroking deeply. You can also make small, deep circles with the thumb tips or use them to press down, hold, then release over deep muscle tissue.

THE ESSENTIAL MASSAGE

Essential oils need to be diluted with a carrier oil before they are massaged into skin. The basic recipe should be:

FOR A BODY MASSAGE
15 drops essential oil
in 60ml (2fl oz/12 tsps) carrier oil

FOR A FACE / FOOT MASSAGE
5 drops of essential oil
in 30ml (1fl oz/6 tsps) carrier oil

Stick to these recipes as it is best to mix only as much as you need each time, so that the vital ingredients stay fresh and uncontaminated. If you make more than you need, store any leftovers out of direct sunlight in a tightly stoppered dark glass bottle.

As to as how much oil is enough for each massage, you need to apply enough to make your hands slip but not slide. Start with a small amount of warm oil and spread it on skin with smooth, flowing, rhythmic strokes, adding more to your hands as they start to drag over skin.

The best carrier oils to give enough slip for massage are sweet almond, sunflower or safflower. These are ideal for both body or face, but if you want to treat a particular type of complexion or skin problem as you massage, use one of the carrier oils specifically for facial skin care (see Best Oils for the Face, page 86).

When preparing your oils, first measure out the carrier then add the essential oil, drop by drop, and shake or stir to blend. In general you should use no more than three essential oils at a time for massage, as any more will only mean the individual aromas fight each other rather than blending together.

HOW TO COMBINE OILS

When it comes to massage, you can use a single oil or mix two or three together. The best essential oils for a single-scented massage are shown right.

When it comes to combining essential oils for massage, the more scented they are the more sensual the massage will be. Touch is even more relaxing with the right aroma to refresh or restore both body and mind. This means many of the most therapeutic oils are left out of the following recipes, because although they might do you good, when it comes to massage for pleasure it must smell good as well. However, if you

---

Best Aromatic Oils

bergamot
geranium
lavender
neroli
orange
rose
ylang-ylang
•

Best Therapeutic Oils

chamomile
(insomnia, stress, tension)
•

eucalyptus
(colds, aching muscles)
•

mimosa
(cheering, anti-depressant)
•

peppermint
(invigorating, energising)
•

rosemary
(mental fatigue, headache)
•

clary sage
(PMT, fatigue, depression)
•

sandalwood
(sensual, sedative, mellow)

need a purely therapeutic massage, look back to the chart of essential oil properties (see page 50) to help you make your choice.

Remember, don't shower or bath for two hours after an aromatherapy massage, so the essential oils have a chance to be totally absorbed. Here are some of the best oils for each of the five massages in this chapter.

RELAXING BACK MASSAGE

The back is one of the best bits of the body to massage , since it has such a tangle of muscles and nerves that it responds dramatically to the right touch. It also is a large, smooth space that is ideal for spreading oil and learning strokes (for a step-by-step back massage, see page 112). Here is a selection of the best aromatherapy oils to use.

Best Oils for Back Massage

bergamot	lavender
eucalyptus	orange
frankincense	petitgrain

BEST COMBINATIONS

RELAXING MASSAGE
7 drops lavender and 4 drops each rose and mimosa in 60ml (2fl oz/12 tsps) sunflower oil

---

ENERGISING MASSAGE
6 drops bergamot, 5 drops peppermint and 2 drops of lemon in 60ml (2fl oz/12 tsps) sweet almond oil

---

WARMING WINTER RUB
6 drops frankincense, 5 drops eucalyptus and 4 drops pine in 60ml (2fl oz/12 tsps) sunflower oil

---

INVIGORATING SUMMER RUB
6 drops orange, 5 drops lemongrass and 4 drops rosemary in 60ml (2fl oz/12 tsps) sweet almond oil

---

FOR BACKACHE
6 drops each lavender and eucalyptus and 3 drops lemon in 60ml (2fl oz/12 tsps) safflower oil

---

FOR TENSE MUSCLES
8 drops lavender, 5 drops petitgrain and 2 drops basil in 60ml (2fl oz/12 tsps) sunflower oil

---

THE THINKER'S MASSAGE

Too much thinking, worrying, concentration or anxiety all end up on the poor old head and shoulders. A face, neck and scalp massage (see page 115) not only relieves the tight, tense muscles, but also puts the evaporating essential oils right under your nose, so they get to work on the over-tired, overwrought mind by the most direct route. Some of the best aromatherapy combinations for the neck up include:

Best Oils for Head Massage

bergamot	neroli
jasmine	orange
lavender	rose

BEST COMBINATIONS

RELAXING MASSAGE
3 drops each rose, geranium and lavender in 30ml (1fl oz/6 tsps) sweet almond oil

ENERGISING MASSAGE
3 drops bergamot and 1 drop each of geranium and peppermint in 30ml (1fl oz/6 tsps) sweet almond oil

FOR TENSE MUSCLES
2 drops each petitgrain and lavender and 1 drop basil in 30ml (1fl oz/6 tsps) sweet almond oil

FOR A HAIR TONIC
3 drops lavender and 1 drop each rosemary and bay in 30ml (1fl oz/6 tsps) sweet almond oil

TO GO TO SLEEP
3 drops sandalwood and 2 drops of chamomile in 30ml (1fl oz/6 tsps) sweet almond oil

FOR A HEADACHE
2 drops each rose and lavender and 1 drop chamomile in 30ml (1fl oz/6 tsps) sunflower oil

ENERGISING BODY RUB

The over-worked, over-stressed under-exercised body blossoms with a daily top-to-toe wake-up massage (see page 118). It not only leaves you energised and raring to go, but it also helps get rid of tense muscles, cellulite and early-morning aches and pains. The best oils that all add to the stimulation are:

Best Oils for Energising Body Rub	
bergamot	orange
lavender	peppermint
lemon	petitgrain

BEST COMBINATIONS

ENERGISING MASSAGE
5 drops each petitgrain, orange and bergamot in 60ml (2fl oz/12 tsps) sunflower oil

FOR TIGHT MUSCLES
5 drops pine, 7 drops lavender and 3 drops eucalyptus in 60ml (2fl oz/12 tssp) sweet almond oil

FOR CELLULITE
4 drops each rosemary and lemon and 9 drops geranium in 60ml (2fl oz/12 tsps) sweet almond oil

FOR WINTER
7 drops lavender and 4 drops each peppermint and myrrh in 60ml (2fl oz/12 tsps) sunflower oil

FOR SUMMER
6 drops lavender, 5 drops orange and 4 drops peppermint in 60ml (2fl oz/12 tsps) sweet almond oil

FOR MENTAL ALERTNESS
6 drops bergamot and 4 drops peppermint in 60ml (2fl oz/12 tsps) sweet almond oil

THE SOOTHING FOOT MASSAGE

The feet take more abuse than any other part of the body. Reward them with a gentle, soothing massage, to spread pleasure throughout your body.

Best Oils for Soothing Foot Massage	
citronella	lemon
geranium	peppermint
lavender	rosemary

BEST COMBINATIONS

RELAXING MASSAGE
3 drops lavender and 2 drops geranium
in 30ml (1fl oz/6 tsps) sunflower oil

REFRESHING MASSAGE
2 drops each citronella and peppermint and 1 drop
lemon in 30ml (1fl oz/6 tsps) sunflower oil

AROMATIC MASSAGE
2 drops each lavender, rose and geranium
in 30ml (1fl oz/6 tsps) sunflower oil

FOR ACHING FEET
3 drops eucalyptus and 2 drops chamomile
in 30ml (1fl oz/6 tsps) sunflower oil

FOR EXCESSIVE SWEATING
5 drops lemongrass
in 30ml (1fl oz/6 tsps) sunflower oil

FOR FUNGAL INFECTIONS
3 drops tea-tree and 2 drops of geranium
in 30ml (1fl oz/6 tsps) sunflower oil

BEST COMBINATIONS

FOR DRY COMPLEXIONS
3 drops rose and 2 drops neroli
in 30ml (1 fl oz/6 tsps) apricot kernel oil

FOR OILY COMPLEXIONS
2 drops each geranium and lavender and 1 drop
bergamot in 30ml (1 fl oz/6 tsps) sunflower oil

YOUNG SKIN (UNDER 40)
3 drops geranium and 2 drops orange
in 30ml (1 fl oz/6 tsps) sweet almond oil

MATURE SKIN (OVER 40)
2 drops each neroli and lavender and 1 drop myrrh
in 30ml (1 fl oz/6 tsps) wheatgerm oil

FOR SUMMER
2 drops each rose and violet and 1 drop geranium
in 30ml (1 fl oz/6 tsps) sunflower oil

FOR WINTER
2 drops each myrrh and sandalwood
in 30ml (1 fl oz/6 tsps) wheatgerm oil

THE ANTI-WRINKLE MASSAGE

An aromatherapy massage takes the stress marks off your face by soothing the anxiety and irritability that cause frowns as it treats the skin itself. It also reduces fine lines and dehydration, and stimulates cell turnover.

Best Oils for Anti-wrinkle Massage

geranium	neroli
lavender	orange
myrrh	rose

Regenerating Oils
Some essences, such as lavender, can encourage the growth of new skin cells. This is why they are so effective in treating injuries such as burns, as well as in preserving a healthy looking skin which is soft to the touch.

111

RELAXING BACK MASSAGE

The best position for a back massage is lying face down on a well-padded
floor or firm mattress with a rolled towel or small pillow under the upper chest,
so the head and neck are relaxed in the face-down position.
Keep the room warm and the light subdued.

Before you begin, warm your hands and warm the aromatherapy massage oil by
standing the containing in hot water for a couple of minutes.
The more times you repeat each stroke the more relaxing it becomes, so use the
instructions here as a guide only for the minimum amount of movements.
And feel free to throw in your own special touches.

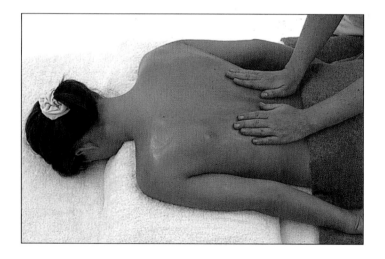

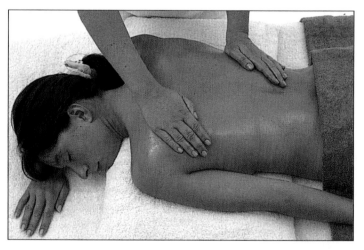

1 Place your palms flat, with hands on the lower back about
2 inches out from the spine. Slide them up to the top of the
back, out over the shoulders and down again to the start. The
heaviest stroke is pushing up towards the heart, with a light
stroke down. Use it to warm and spread the oil and feel for
tension or tender spots in the back. Keep a soothing, regular
rhythm going for several minutes, then spread fingers wide on
the upward stroke only, pressing in with the tips, for a slightly
deeper variation.

2 With palms flat half way up the spine, gently slide your
hands apart the length of the back, so one ends at the base
of the spine and the other between the shoulder blades. Repeat
several times. Then from the same start position, slide hands
diagonally across the torso so one ends on a hip and the other
on the opposite shoulder. Repeat, both ways. Each movement
should be one long, firm stroke to loosen and stretch muscles,
holding skin taught at the end for a few seconds before releasing
the tension.

3 ▶ Repeat the stroke from step 1, but this time, when you get to the top, slide your hands over the shoulders, bending your fingertips down to the collarbones, and on the downward stroke, pull the shoulder muscle at the base of the neck firmly back. Repeat. Place your hands under the hip, fingers down, and pull upwards from the side of the body towards the spine, one hand after the other in a continuous movement. Work up one side of the torso, across the top of the shoulders and down the other side to the opposite hip.

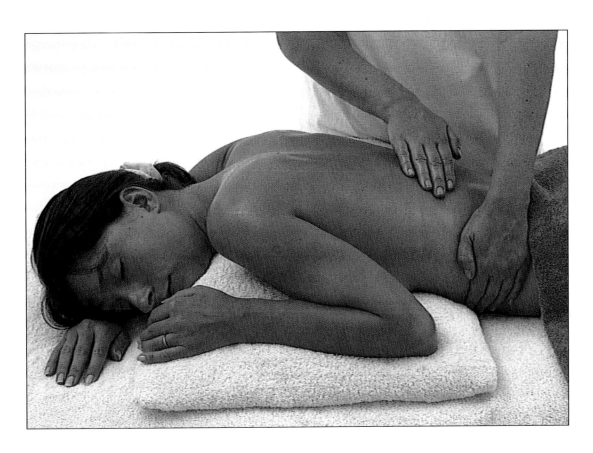

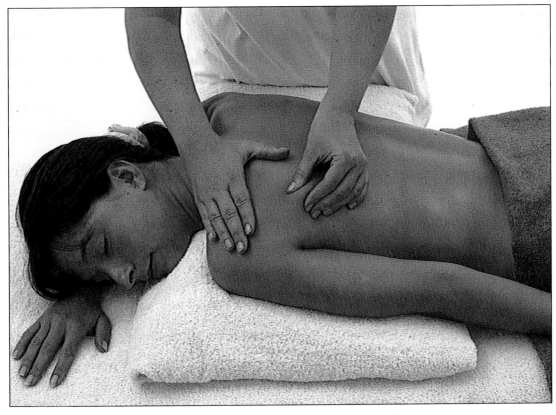

4 ◀ Moving to the upper back, place palms flat on either side of the spine above the waist and push them up to the neck, out around each shoulder and back to the start position. Keep the stroke flowing, then do smaller circles using fingertip rather than palm-pressure around and over each shoulder blade. Then knead the upper back and sides of the neck – place your hands flat, fingers together with thumbs wide, then use your thumbs to push flesh up to the fingers, moving your hands as you go.

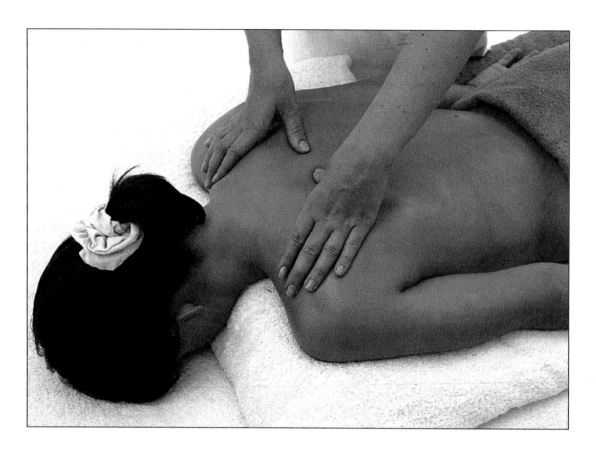

5 ◀ Moving to the lower back, repeat a few sweeping strokes from step 1. Then place one thumb on either side of the spine about an inch out, and gently push down with the thumb pads for a count of five, then relax, to release the small spinal support muscles. Keep doing this, moving up the back to the top of the neck. Repeat from the bottom, this time making tiny circles with each thumb on either side of the spine up to the neck. Finish by running your fingertips firmly up and down over the same area.

6 ▶ Now repeat the smooth, flowing strokes from step 1 again, over the entire back. Then use your fingertips to make circular movements from the base of the back up to the neck. Finally, do a raking movement all over the back – bend your fingers so only the pads make contact, then make short, firm stroking movements, pulling towards you. Start raking at the neck and work down to the hips, so one hand follows the other in a continuous flow. Repeat several times, reducing the amount of pressure so you finish with a light, slow movement.

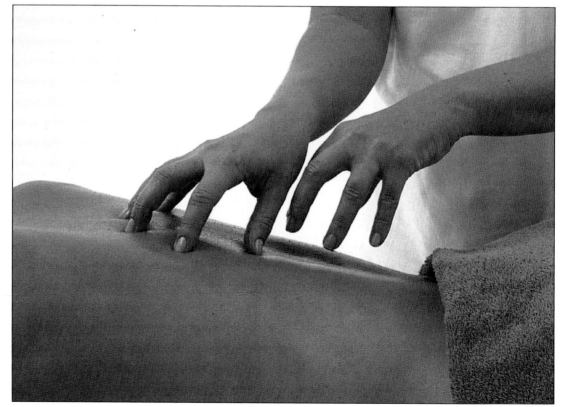

THE THINKER'S MASSAGE

A face, neck and scalp massage will lift a great weight off tired or tense
shoulders. Start by sitting comfortably on an upright chair in front of a table, wearing
an off-the-shoulder top or a towel wrapped under your arms for warmth.
Make sure your aromatherapy oil is also warm, and close to hand.

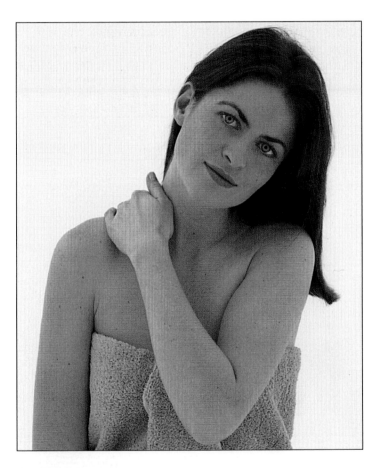

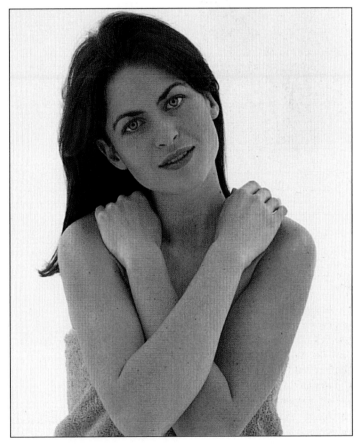

1 Keeping your back straight, slowly bend your neck to one side as far as is comfortable, so your ear is parallel with your shoulder. Hold the stretch for a count of five and feel it pulling up the side of the neck. Straighten slowly and repeat on the other side. With your head upright, place your left hand palm down on the top of your right arm. With a downward pressure, stroke firmly across the top of the shoulder and up the side of the neck to the ear. Repeat ten times, then change hands and repeat on the other side.

2 Bend your elbows and place your hands palm down back over your shoulders, on either side of the neck, with the heel of your hand on your collarbone and fingers stretching down your back. Press firmly into the shoulder muscle, so it is pinched between your fingers and palm, and at the same time, drop your head backwards. Hold for a count of ten then slowly raise the head and release the hands. Repeat. In the same starting position, drop your head first down to the left side for a count of five, then over and down to the right, while you pinch into the shoulder muscle. Repeat.

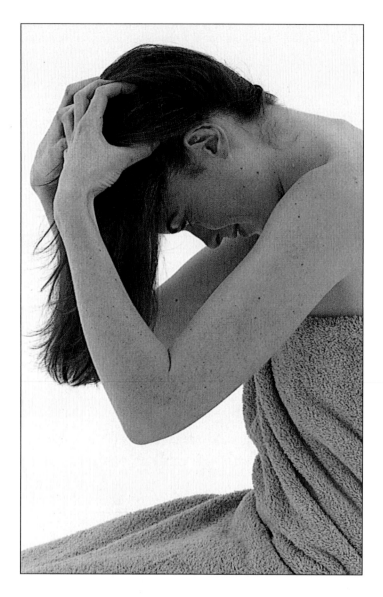

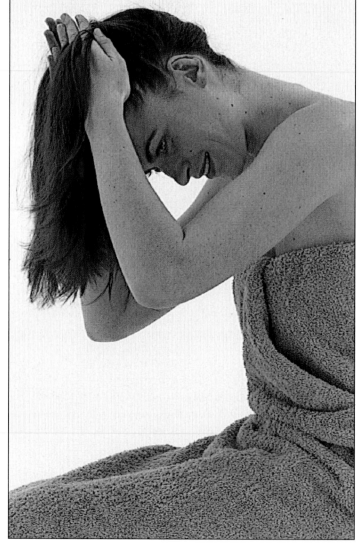

3 ◀ Bend your neck forward and place your fingertips back over the shoulder muscles as in step 2. Knead the muscle by pressing in with firm fingers and gradually work up each side of the neck from the nape to the skull. Then use the first two fingers of each hand to make small circles from the top of the neck out along the base of the skull to each ear. With your head still bent forward, place your right hand palm down over the nape of your neck and do a slow, firm, upward-pulling stroke from the nape up to the crown of the head, with one hand following after the other.

4 ▶ Spread your fingertips across the top of your forehead along the hairline from ear to ear. Keeping fingers bent but stiff, press them gently into the scalp and make small, firm circular movements so the scalp itself rotates. Gradually move, inch by inch, back up to the crown of the head. Repeat working from the nape of the neck up to the crown. Then pick up tiny sections of hair close to the root between each thumb and index finger and tug at the hair, quickly and firmly several times. Repeat all over the head to stimulate the circulation and relax the scalp.

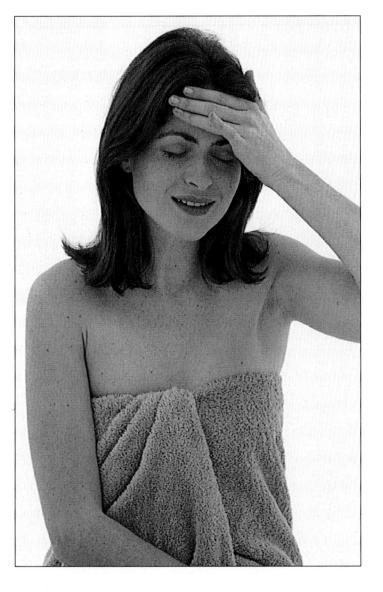

5 ◄ Lean forward and rest your elbows on a table. Place the heel of each hand over an eye and relax downwards, holding for a count of ten and breathing deeply. Straighten the first three fingers of your right hand and place them across your forehead. Stroke slowly and firmly from the bridge of the nose up between the brows to the hair line. Repeat five times. Using your first two fingers, gently press in and stroke from your inner to outer brows. Repeat five times. With one hand on either side of the face, do a firm, very slow, palm stroke from the ears, over the temples, forehead and into the hair. Repeat.

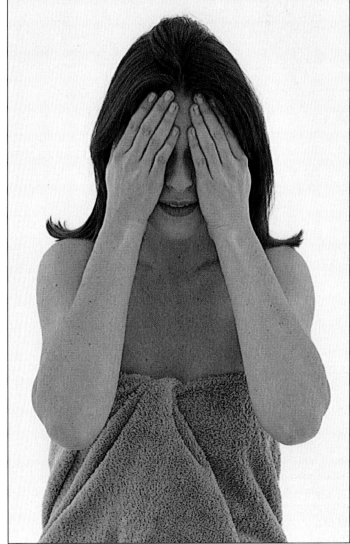

6 ► Using the tips of your first two fingers, make small circles over the whole face, from the jaw, up the cheeks, over the temples and along the hairline to the middle of the forehead. Repeat with a slow, firm, palm stroke. Then, placing the hands with palms over the cheek bones and fingers over the forehead, gently press into the contours of your face and hold for a count of ten. With one palm across your forehead and the other across the back of your neck, press in for a count of ten. With one hand over an ear on either side of your head, press in and hold.

THE ENERGISING BODY RUB

This massage takes ten minutes first thing in the morning, but brings rewards that last a lifetime. The whole sequence is done standing up, and you only need a chair or the side of a bath or bed to rest your foot on in step 1. Make sure you have plenty of aromatherapy massage oil to hand before you begin.

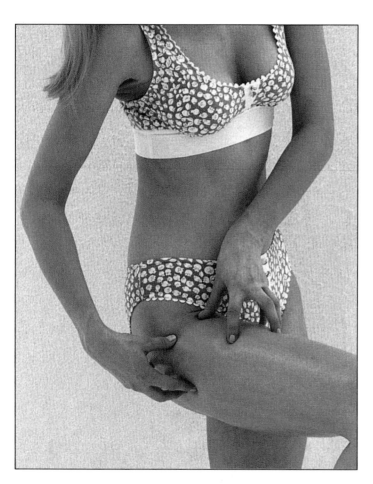

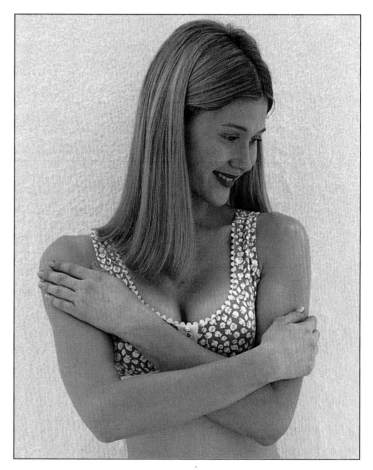

1 Standing, with one foot up on a chair so the knee is at a right angle, do firm, upward palm strokes with one hand following the other from ankle to knee. Do the front, back and sides of each leg. Straighten the leg to stroke from the knee to thigh top, front, back and sides. Then repeat, this time using stiff, bent fingers to rake the legs in an upwards stroke, but have the hands in unison so one is raking the front as the other does the back of the leg. Use the same stroke up both sides of each leg, too.

2 With arms loose at your sides, shake your hands, so they are floppy from the elbow down, as if you're shaking water off. Stretch straight arms up above your head, out to the sides parallel with shoulders, and downwards to toes. Bend your right arm so the hand is at your shoulder, and using your left hand, palm down, wrap your fingers around the top of the arm and do one firm stroke down the arm to the elbow, then up the forearm from elbow to wrist. Continue the stroke, with the thumb pressing into the palm and fingers wrapped around the back of the hand, right up to the fingertips. Repeat on both arms.

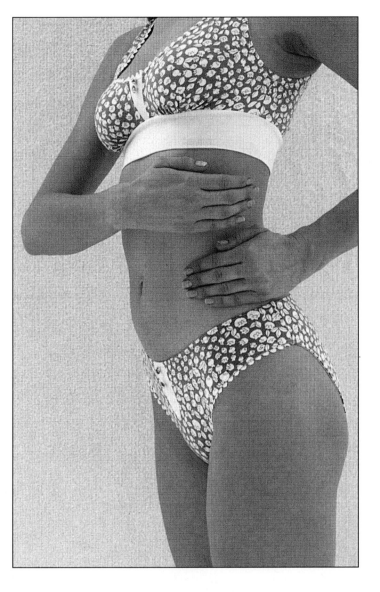

3 ◀ Shape your hands into relaxed fists and use them to pummel the tops of the thighs and buttocks by bouncing them off flesh in a rapid, drumming movement. Do a waist stroke starting on your right side, with your right hand over the the hip, fingers pointing to the navel and left hand over the waist, fingers pointing to back. Stroke one hand after the other in a firm, rhythmic upwards motion from hip to rib. Do 20 strokes in total, then repeat on the other side of the waist. Finally, do the same rhythmic stroke up the tummy, from groin to ribcage.

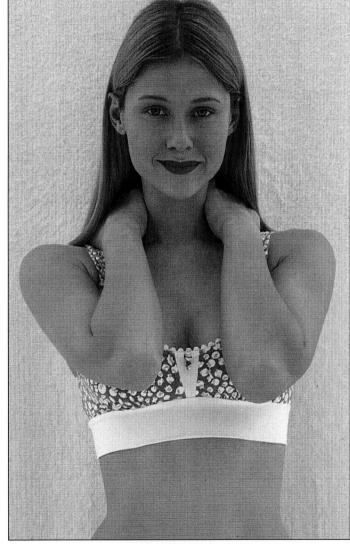

4 ▶ Place your hands up on each shoulder, with a thumb below and index fingers above the collarbone, then pinch and squeeze the bone, working from the shoulder in towards the chest. With palms down, place one hand back over each shoulder top, then pinch and knead the muscle between the fingertips and heel of each hand. Then wrap one hand palm down across the nape of the neck and as you relax the head slightly backwards, pinch and knead the neck muscles.

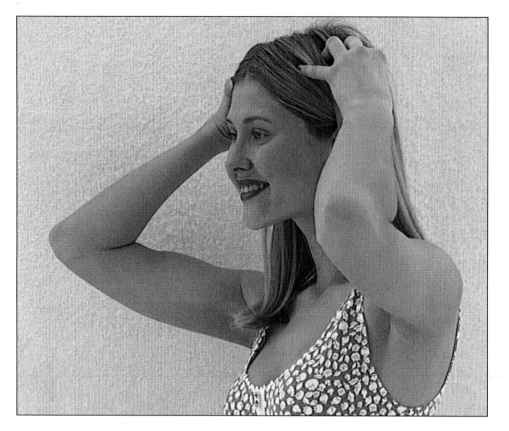

5 ◄ With arms to your sides, stretch and hold your shoulders, by rounding them forwards (head down), backwards (head back), up towards your ears and down (head straight). Hold each stretch for a count of ten before relaxing. Repeat the shoulders forward and backwards movement, but this time with straight arms out at shoulder height. Then shake your head vigorously as if you are shaking water from your hair. With stiff, straight fingers, massage is small circles all over your scalp as if you are shampooing your hair.

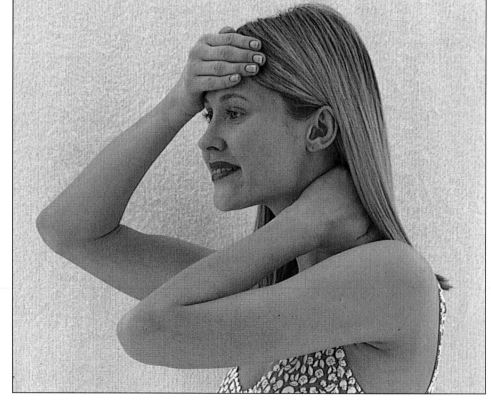

6 ► Bend your arms at the elbows and with floppy, relaxed hands, shake them vigorously as if you're flicking water off them. Then with one hand following the other in a smooth, flowing rhythm, stroke palms down from your brows up the forehead and into your hair for a count of 60. Finish off with a firm head press: place your left hand, palm down, on forehead and right hand palm down across the nape of your neck. Push both hands inwards and hold for a count of 15. Relax and repeat.

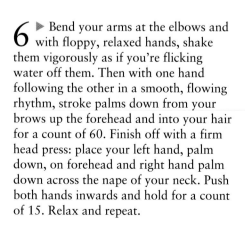

SOOTHING FOOT MASSAGE

The foot massage, with its soothing aromatherapy soak beforehand,
will make you feel better from toe to top and is guaranteed to put a spring back in
your step. Sit in an upright seat with cushions for comfort and finish off
the massage by stretching out flat for ten minutes with feet propped
higher than your head.

You may use the same essential oils for the footbath and massage, or use a purely
therapeutic one for the bath and more sensual oils for the stroking afterwards. Spend
as long as you can on each step, with plenty of extra repeats.

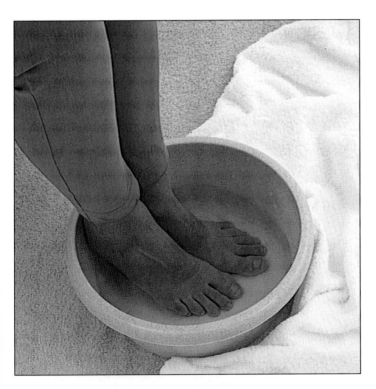

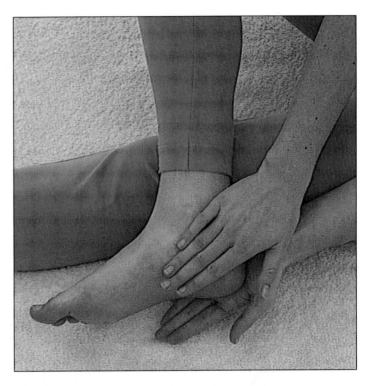

1 Start sitting comfortably with a plastic basin or large bowl of hot water on the floor. Make sure towels, essential oils and your aromatherapy massage oil are all to hand. Put four drops of essential oils for every 4 litres (1 gallon) of water in the bowl and soak both feet. After ten minutes, start massaging one foot while it is still damp, so essential oils absorb better, and leave the other foot in the basin. To massage, sit with one leg bent at the knee and cross it so the calf is resting across the thigh of the other leg.

2 With the palms of your hands, sandwich the foot and do a fast, friction rub, using lots of oil and doing a sawing movement back and forwards across the foot. Start with one hand under the arch and the other across the top of the foot. Then move hands up to sandwich the toes and instep. Finally, do a heel rub by placing palms on either side of the ankle and massaging briskly. This is a good way of boosting the circulation, warming cold feet and relaxing them totally.

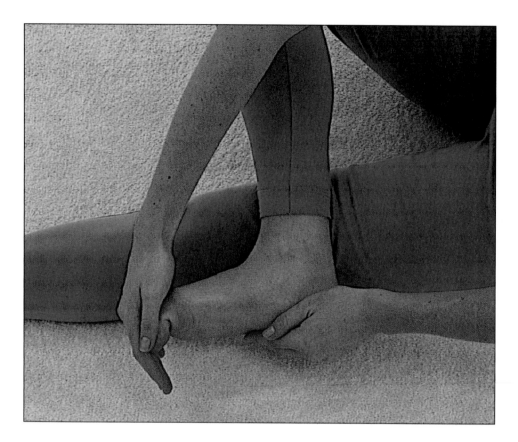

3 ◀ Do a series of foot stretches to loosen tendons and the deep ache of muscles. Hold each stretch for a count of ten. Point your toes and flex them up, hold, then down, hold, and turn your foot to the left, hold, and right, hold. Still pointing your toes, make large, slow circles in the air to rotate the ankle. Then, with your foot resting up on your opposite thigh again, place your hand palm down over the toes with the fingers wrapped over the sole. Keeping your foot straight (i.e. at 90 degree angle to leg), slowly push the toes down to flex and stretch them, and hold. Then gently pull them back towards the foot.

4 ▶ In the same position, use the tips of your thumb and index finger to make quick pinches for several minutes all over the heel of the foot. Then wrap your fingers around the top of the foot with thumbs across the sole, under the arch. Do deep, flowing thumb strokes, one after the other, from the heel to the instep along the arch of the foot. Then use the thumbs to make small circles all over the sole of the foot, in a light, kneading movement.

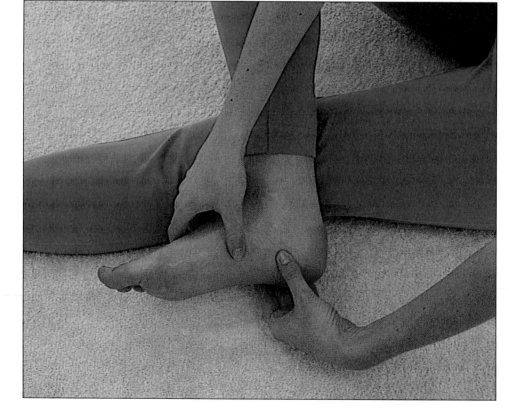

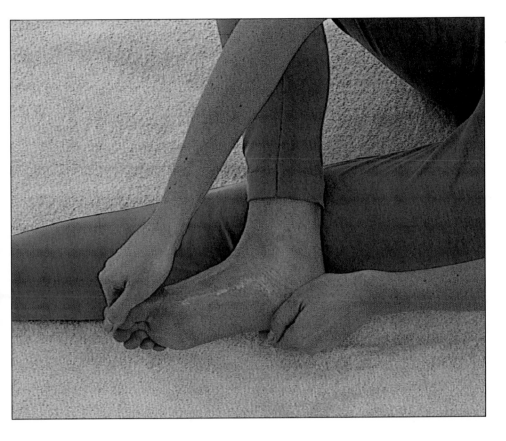

5 ◄ Firmly rub each toe from base to tip, one by one, between your thumb (on top) and index finger (below) for a couple of minutes each. Then do a several deep thumb-strokes up the underside of each toe, by wrapping your fingers across the tops of toes, bending your thumb underneath, and using it to do the firm, slow, pushing in movement. Finally, finish of with a fast friction rub over the toes to warm them and increase blood circulation.

6 ► Use your thumb to knead and rub all around the ankle bone and pinch, using your index finger and thumb, all the way up the tendon at the back of the heel. Repeat the foot stretches from step 3, but this time keep both hands wrapped around your ankle as you point, flex and circle them. Finish off with several full foot-strokes. Place one hand on top of the foot, palm down, the other under the foot, palm up. Start at the toes and with hands working in unison, do a firm, slow pull with hands, following the contours of the foot back up to the ankle.

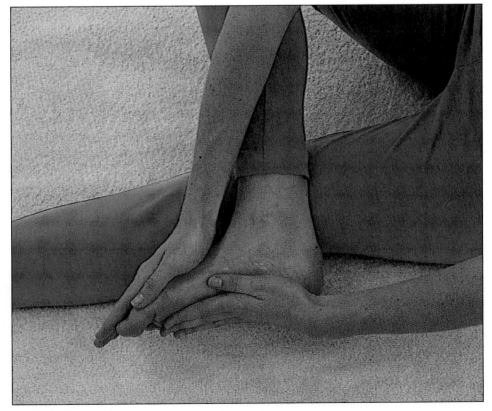

THE ANTI-WRINKLE MASSAGE

Although wrinkles are a sign of a life well-lived, nobody likes to see them appearing on their own face. There are only two things, apart from surgery, that will help keep wrinkles at bay: protecting skin from the sun, and making sure it is well moisturised. Essential oils do the latter better than any other products, since they have a natural affinity with skin and are absorbed into the body.

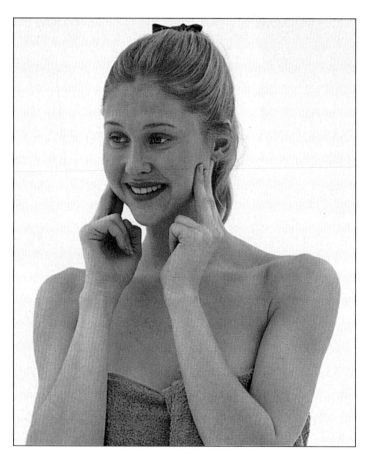

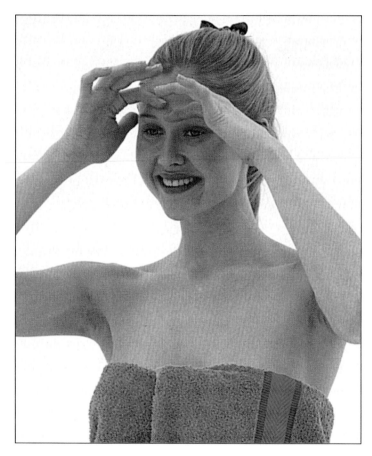

1 Place the first two fingers of each hand under each earlobe, press in gently for a count of six, then slide fingers up the side of the face to the temples. Press in gently for a count of six, then release and make small, gentle circles over the temples with your fingertips. Put your little fingers next to one another on the bridge of the nose and, keeping them stiff and splayed, place the others along each brow, so the index fingers are on the temples. Press in gently, hold for a count of six, then press in again and slide your fingers up the brow into the hairline, pulling skin up as you move, and finish with small circular movements pressing into the scalp. Repeat five times.

2 Stretch your neck by bending your head back and holding for a count of six while you open yokujr eyes wide and raise your eyebrows. With head upright, place your index fingers next to one another on the bridge of the nose and stroke upwards, one after the other, between the brows to the forehead. Every sixth stroke, take one finger out firmly along each brow and press into the temple for a count of three. Repeat several times. Then, using the flat of your hand, palm-stroke up the forehead into the hair, one hand following the other.

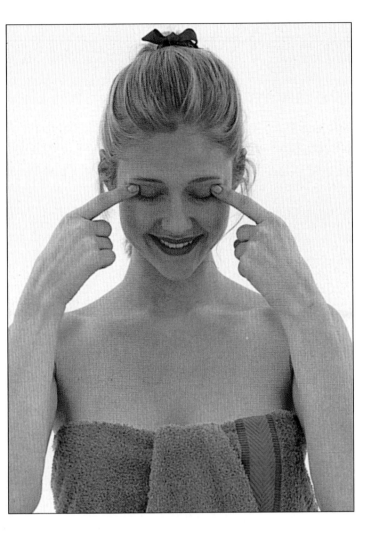

3 ◄ Place each index finger at the outer eye corner, then move them gradually along the undereye, making gentle inward presses for a count of three until you are pressing in on the tear ducts. This is a very light pressure throughout. Repeat on the top eyelid, along the browbone. Don't stretch or drag on the skin, rather press in, lift, then press again. Place the heel of each hand over the eyes and gently press while you relax and count to 20. Finally, screw your eyes tightly closed and hold for a count of five. Then open them wide and roll the eyes in slow circles three times.

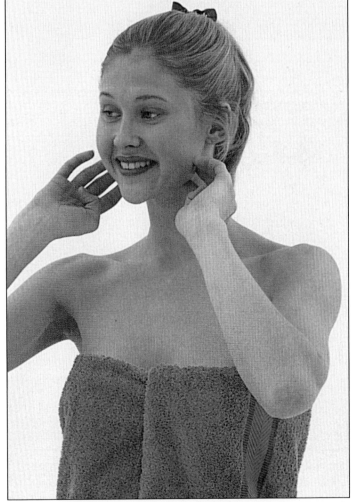

4 ► Stretch the neck by bending the head to one side, hold for a count of ten, then over to the other side and hold. With your head straight, use the backs of the fingertips to stroke from the collarbone up to the chin in a rhythmic, flowing movement. Then, with palms facing up, use the first three fingertips of each hand to do a light, outward flick under the chin, in a rapid drumming motion across the entire jawline from ear to ear. With thumbs and forefingers, lightly pinch along the jawbone from chin out to earlobes. Repeat back to the middle of the chin.

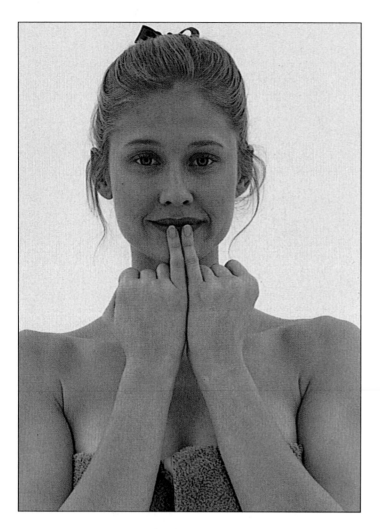

5 ◄ Open your mouth wide and with a relaxed jaw, move your chin to the left, hold for a count of five, then to the right and hold for another five. Place the tips of your little fingers on the middle of your bottom lip, press in, hold for a count of five, then repeat, gradually moving out to the corners of the mouth, then up and over the top lip to the centre of the nose. Repeat as a light stroke. Finish by pressing your palm over your mouth and holding for a count of ten.

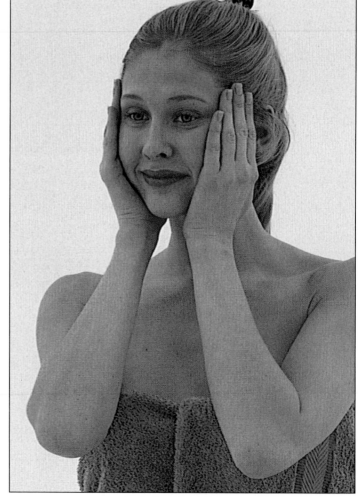

6 ▶ Place the palms of your hands against the sides of your face and stroke with a fast, light touch in an upwards direction to stimulate circulation and bring the colour to your cheeks. Repeat the same stroke, but with a slow, firm stretch upwards. Finish off by pressing the palms of your hands over your face and holding for a count of 20.

INDEX

ACKNOWLEDGEMENTS

(Abbreviations: r = right, l = left, t = top, c = centre, b = below)

Robert Harding Picture Library: page 102.
Image Bank / Stuart Dee: page 1t; / Lou Jones: page 1b; / Weinberg / Clark: page 8; / Manuel Rodriguez:

page 9; / Lawrence Berman: page 10; / Nicholas Foster: page 11t; / Murray Alcosser: page 44.
PWA International: pages 12, 15, 17, 57, 59, 61, 64, 68, 70, 84, 90b, 94.
Spectrum Colour Library: pages 53, 67.

Tony Stone Images: page 11b; / Mike Busselle: page 2-3; / Charles Thatcher: pages 18, 62; / Howard Grey: page 48; / Bruce Ayres: page 58; / Ian O'Leary: page 76; / Ken Fisher: page 98; / John Fortunato: page 100-1.
ZEFA: pages 6, 79, 103.

Every effort has been made to trace the copyright holders and we apologise in advance for any unintentional omissions. We would be pleased to insert the appropriate acknowledgement in any subsequent edition of this publication.